The Effect of Immunological and Non-Immunological Factors on Corneal Graft Survival

MONOGRAPHS IN OPHTHALMOLOGY

P.C. Maudgal and L. Missotten (eds.), Superficial Keratitis. 1981.
ISBN 90-6193-801-5.

P.F.J. Hoyng, Pharmacological Denervation and Glaucoma. A Clinical Trial Report with Guanethidine and Adrenaline in One Eye Drop. 1981.
ISBN 90-6193-802-3.

N.W.H.M. Dekkers, The Cornea in Measles. 1981. ISBN 90-6193-803-1.

P. Leonard and J. Rommel, Lens Implantation – 30 years of progress. 1982.
ISBN 90-6193-804-X.

C.E. van Nouhuys, Dominant Exudative Vitreoretinopathy and Other Vascular Developmental Disorders of the Peripheral Retina. 1982. ISBN 90-6193-805-8.

L. Evens (ed.), Convergent Strabismus. 1982. ISBN 90-6193-806-6.

A. Neetens, A. Löwenthal and J.J. Martin (eds.), The Visual System in Myelin Disorders. 1984. ISBN 90-6193-807-4.

H.J.M. Völker-Dieben, The Effect of Immunological and Non-Immunological Factors on Corneal Graft Survival. 1984. ISBN 90-6193-808-2.

The Effect of Immunological and Non-Immunological Factors on Corneal Graft Survival

A Single Centre Study

by

H.J.M. Völker-Dieben

1984 **DR W. JUNK PUBLISHERS**
a member of the KLUWER ACADEMIC PUBLISHERS GROUP
DORDRECHT / BOSTON / LANCASTER

Distributors

for the United States and Canada: Kluwer Academic Publishers, 190 Old Derby Street, Hingham, MA 02043, USA
for the UK and Ireland: Kluwer Academic Publishers, MTP Press Limited, Falcon House, Queen Square, Lancaster LA1 1RN, England
for all other countries: Kluwer Academic Publishers Group, Distribution Center, P.O. Box 322, 3300 AH Dordrecht, The Netherlands

Library of Congress Cataloging in Publication Data

Völker-Dieben, H. J. M.
The effect of immunological and non-immunological factors on corneal graft survival.

(Monographs in ophthalmology ; 8)
"Reprinted from Documenta Ophthalmologica ; vol. 57, issue 1/2."
Includes bibliographies.
1. Cornea--Transplantation--Addresses, essays, lectures. 2. Cornea--Transplantation--Immunological aspects--Addresses, essays, lectures. 3. Graft rejection --Addresses, essays, lectures. I. Title. II. Series. [DNLM: 1. Cornea--transplantation. 2. Graft Survival. 3. Antigens, Immune Response--analysis. 4. Transplantation Immunology. W1 MO568D v.8 / WW 220 V917e]
RE336.V65 1984 617.7'19 84-14350
ISBN 90-6193-808-2

REPRINTED FROM Documenta Ophthalmologica Volume 57 issue 1/2

ISBN-13: 978-94-009-6568-3 e-ISBN-13: 978-94-009-6566-9
DOI: 10.1007/978-94-009-6566-9

CONTENTS

Abbreviations

A.C.	– Anterior Chamber
C.M.E.	– Cystoid Macular Oedema
C.V.A.	– Cerebro Vascular Accident
H-2	– The major histocompatibility complex in mice. Subdivided in class I loci: K, D and L and class II loci (= I-region) i.g. A and E.
HLA	– Human leucocyte antigen region, the major histocompatibility complex in man. Subdivided in class I loci: A, B and C and class II loci: e.g. D/DR and SB.
H.S.V.	– Herpes Simplex Virus
I.O.L.	– Intraocular Lens
I.O.P.	– Intraocular Pressure
Ir genes	– Immune response genes
M.C.M.	– Malignant Choroidal Melanoma
M.H.C.	– The Major Histocompatibility Complex
P.E.D.	– Primary Endothelial Decompensation (Fuchs' dystrophy)
P.K.P.	– Penetrating Keratoplasties
P.L.	– Product Limit
R.R.	– Relative Risk
S.E.	– Standard Errors
S.E.D.	– Secondary Endothelial Decompensation (bullous keratopathy)
T.F.T.	– Trifluor Thymidine (antiviral eye drops

CHAPTER 1

Introduction*

'The clinical importance of corneal grafting lies in the fact that successful transplantation can restore excellent sight to persons suffering from corneal blindness' (Jones 1973).

In 1831, the possibility of a successful corneal transplantation was considered as 'certainly one of the most audacious fantasies, and it would be the highest reward of surgery if this operation succeeded' (Dieffenbach 1831). One hundred twenty five years later, Thomas reported that 'it was universally accepted that the results of keratoplasty are good' (Thomas 1955). At that time the level of clear grafts was around 50% (Stansbury 1949, Owens et al. 1949, Ciotola 1949, Roberts 1950, Löhlein 1950). In 1980, Bloomfield reported that 'corneal transplantation enjoys a high success rate because the avascularity of the cornea and the absence of lymphatic drainage in this area bestow a considerably degree of immunological privilege'. That hypothesis had been presented as early as 1965 by Nelken. Sanfilippo (1982) classified penetrating keratoplasty as 'a routine and somewhat benign procedure'. In just over 150 years, a most audacious fantasy has been transformed into a routine procedure.

Although corneas are one of the most successful transplanted organs in transplantation surgery, nevertheless corneal transplantation presents problems similar to those seen in other types of organ allografting, namely surgical complications and graft rejection. The progressive refinements in surgical techniques, the introduction of surgical microscopes, continuous monofilament nylon sutures and the preservation of the integrity of the donor cornea endothelium during transplantation have improved the prognosis for corneal graft survival considerably. By 1976, just before the implementation of HLA matching 71.5% clear grafts were observed on one year post transplantation in our center (chapter 5). Technical improvements have enabled ophthalmic surgeons to graft less favourable cases. These cases are those characterized by corneas which may have lost their so called immunological privilege because of severe vascular ingrowth. Consequently, allograft rejection remains the ultimate limitation to corneal transplantation. The number of patients with graft rejections increases quantitatively in time because of the cumulation of these patients during the years.

The prognosis of repeated grafts is significantly less favourable than that of first grafts (Batchelor et al. 1976 and chapter 5). Arentsen et al. (1976) and Smith et al. (1980) reported increasing percentages of regrafts in the period between 1941 and 1978.

Motivation

The severe psychological trauma experienced by patients who lose their visual acuity, after having had it restored for a few months with their initially clear corneal grafts, prompted us to investigate the possible causes of graft rejection with the aim of reducing their numbers (See colour plate 4, c and d). Thanks to the help of the Department of Immunohaematology (chairman Prof. Dr. J.J. van Rood) and financial support from several societies for the blind, we were able to start a pilot study in 1976 to investigate the effect of prospective HLA-A and -B matching on corneal graft survival. Two years later a grant from the Netherlands Organization for Applied Scientic Research (TNO) (GO 77-8) made a more extensive study possible. Although our initial goal was to study the effect of prospective HLA-A and -B matching on corneal graft survival, we soon realized that this was impossible without also considering other factors which influence corneal graft survival, i.e. vascularisation of the recipient cornea, previous graft failure and the initial corneal disease.

HLA: Major histocompatibility complex of man (MHC)

In 1946, Medawar demonstrated the homology between leukocytes and tissue antigens in rabbits (Medawar 1946). Eight years later the formation of leukoagglutinins following blood transfusions was reported by Miescher and Fauconnet (1954), Dausset (1954) and Spielmann (1955). Four years later Payne and Rolfs (1958) and Van Rood (1958) simultaneously reported the formation of leukoagglutinins following pregnancies. In the ensuing 25 years, microlymphocytotoxicity assays, introduced by Terasaki and McClelland (1964) have replaced these early macro leukoagglutination techniques. The rapidity and large scale standardization of those techniques (Van Rood 1976 and 1979), the introduction of a systematic approach to the analysis of their serologic results (Van Rood 1962) and eight International Histocompatibility Workshops and Conferences have resulted in the definition of more than 80 specificities in the human Major Histocompatiblity Complex. Amos 1968, Bodmer et al. 1966, Ceppelini et al. 1967, Dausset et al. 1965, Kissmeyer-Nielsen et al. 1968, Van Rood et al. 1965 were responsible for marking out the genetics of HLA (Histocompatibility Locus A.).

HLA is located on the short arm of chromosome six. Its genes are organized into at least 5 tightly linked loci, A, B, C, D, DR; each with multiple alleles which code for different tissue antigens. Besides those officially recognized loci, there is increasing evidence for the existence of additional loci: MB and SB (see fig. 1) (Duquesnoy et al. 1980 and Shaw et al. 1980). Since transplantation does not occur in nature, excluding 'the foetal allograft', the reasons for the presentation of the MHC's throughout phylogeny must be sought in other areas. The linkage of H-2 to susceptibility to viral leukemogenesis in mice, the significant associations between HLA-antigens in various diseases, e.g. Ankylosing spondylitis and Insulin Dependent Diabetes Mellitus and the report by De Vries et al. (1979) for a possible role for genes within the MHC for the genetic control of survival in epidemics are all suggestive of an important function of the MHC's. There is an increasing evidence that class II molecules (DR, D, SB, MT and MB) of the MHC may be immune response (Ir) genes and that class I molecules (A, B and C) may also be involved in the immuneresponse (Klein et al. 1981, Benacerraf 1981).

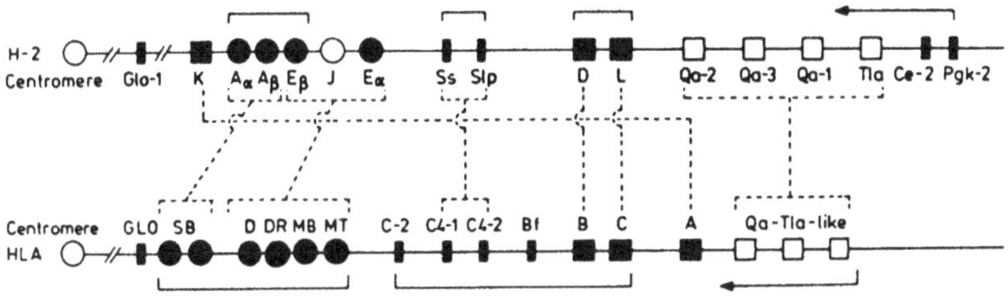

Figure 1. The major histocompatibility complex: a schematic representation of the organization on the chromosome of the loci composing the mouse (H-2) and human (HLA) regions. In mice the MCH is situated on chromosome 17, and in man on chromosome 6.

Presumed homologies between loci of H-2 and HLA are connected by dotted lines. The different loci are named by capitals. Closed squares represent class I loci. In mice these are K, D and L, in man A, B and C. Closed circles represent class II loci. In mice these are A and E, in man DR and less well defined D, SB, MT and MB.

Loci coding for complement components (class III: in mice Ss and Slp, in man C2, C3 and Bf) and enzyme coding loci (GLO = glyoxylase, Ce-2 = liver catalase and Pgk-2 = phosphoglycerate kinase-2) in/or closely linked to the MHC are represented by bars).

Open squares represent a second family of class I loci which code for class I products with a distinct tissue distribution, in man they are as yet not well defined.

From: An approach to study the genetic control of the antigen-specific immune response in man Evert J. Hensen (1982).

Objectives

The studies in this thesis may be divided into three sections:

Section I: **Donor corneas from eyes containing a malignant choroidal melanoma;**
This section considers the consequences of using corneas from living donors with malignant choroidal melanoma for transplantation;

Section II: **Factors which may influence corneal graft surival;**
This section addresses itself to the effect of immunological and nonimmunological factors on the survival of corneal allografts;

Section III: **HLA and ABO associations in eye diseases;**
This section presents the results of studies on the distributions of the HLA antigens in different subsets of transplanted patients and donors.

Section I

Living donors, i.e. those who provided corneas from eyes enucleated because of serious diseases in the posterior part of the bulbus, have had a key position in corneal transplantation in two different time periods. When corneal transplantation was started in The Netherlands in 1939, the only source of donor material were corneas from eyes enucleated because of serious diseases in the posterior part of the bulbus but with clear corneas. In fact, the primary and almost exclusive source of donor material was corneas from eyes enucleated because of malignant choroidal melanoma (MCM). The consequences of the use of those donor corneas with particular attention to the possible transmission of tumour cells to the recipient by the graft were studied. Since 22 corneal grafts were performed between 1939 and 1948 in the Leyden University Eye Clinic with that type of donor material, these patients had in principal a sufficiently long follow-up period so that the possible influence on their causes of death could be studied (chapter 3).

In 1976 when tissue typing for the purpose of matching was applied to corneal graft donors, the results were more reliable with blood samples from living donors than with those from cadaveric donors. For that reason, we used just as in 1939 donor corneas from eyes of living donors, enucleated because of MCM. The aim of the study was to investigate the survival of donor corneas from eyes enucleated because of MCM versus the graft survival of corneas obtained postmortem from donors with systemic malignancies in the same period (chapter 4).

Section II

In section II non-immunological and immunological factors which influence corneal graft survival are described. In contrast to kidney transplantation where a complete organ is transplanted and connected to the vascular system of the recipient, a corneal graft consists only of the central part of the donor cornea. The graft has to be sutured to the periferal part of the diseased host cornea. Moreover, the possibility for a temporary functional replacement of the organ, like dialysis before kidney transplantation is, of course, impossible before corneal transplantation. This situation forces surgeons to perform corneal grafts à chaud in actively inflamed herpes keratitis corneas, in those with imminent perforation or in those with an already perforated descemetocele.

A great advantage in studies on corneal transplants is the possibility for direct observation of the transplanted cornea. Biomicroscopy provides the ophthalmologist with detailed clinical information with regard to the clarity and thus the vitality and general condition of the graft. For instance, leucocyte infiltrations are directly visible. However in contrast to the situation in nephrology it is impossible to obtain biopsy material from a rejected corneal graft.

The diagnosis of graft rejection is a clinical decision. The criteria for this diagnosis, as summed up during the Ciba Foundation Symposium on corneal graft failure held in 1972 (see Ciba Foundation Symposium, 1973) are as follows: 'the unequivocal diagnosis of an allograft reaction can be made when at least 10 days after a first transplantation a previously clear graft in a quiet eye rapidly develops oedema with signs of inflammation in the anterior segment including ciliary flush, with cells and usually a slight flare in the anterior chamber and when the area of oedema in the graft moves across the cornea in the wake of an endothelial line (Khodadoust rejection line)'. These criteria for an allograft reaction after a first graft have been used also for the diagnosis of an allograft rejection in repeated grafts. The function of a corneal graft cannot be measured solely by the assessment of the visual acuity, since an irregular anterior curvature with corneal astigmatism, cataract formation, abnormal structures in the vitreous and finally retinal and optic nerve diseases influence the visual acuity. Consequently, the optical clarity of the graft is, therefore, a better criterium when we are considering the longterm survival of the graft. However, optical clarity is a subjective criterium and no objective and reproducable methods for analysing the optical clarity are available. Fully aware of the unavoidable subjectivity in the evaluation of graft survival, a decision was made that only one ophthalmologist among the two who performed the transplants would fill in the corneal graft follow-up forms. Those forms were designed for this study and were not changed during the period of the study (fig. 2). Personal information and cell numbers from recipient and donor were recorded. The

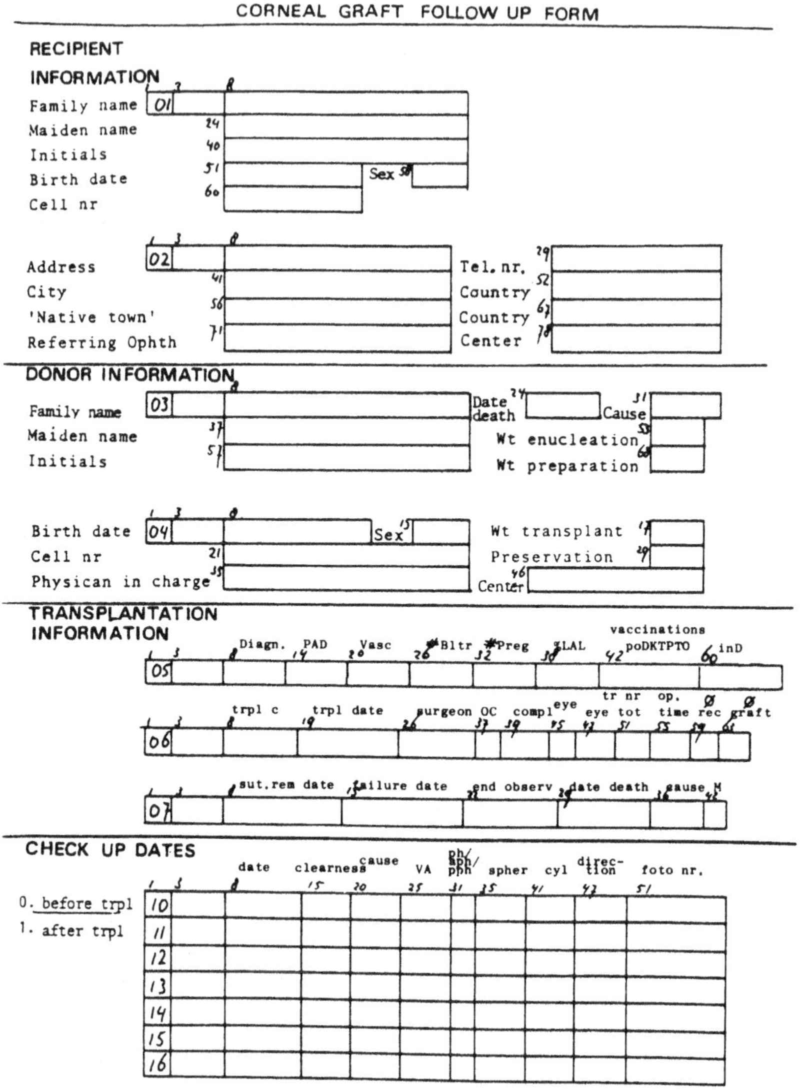

CORNEAL GRAFT FOLLOW UP FORM

RECIPIENT INFORMATION

Family name 01
Maiden name
Initials
Birth date — Sex
Cell nr

Address 02 — Tel. nr.
City — Country
'Native town' — Country
Referring Ophth — Center

DONOR INFORMATION

Family name 03 — Date death — Cause
Maiden name — Wt enucleation
Initials — Wt preparation

Birth date 04 — Sex — Wt transplant
Cell nr — Preservation
Physican in charge — Center

TRANSPLANTATION INFORMATION

05 — Diagn. — PAD — Vasc — #Bltr — #Preg — LAL — vaccinations poDKTPTO — inD

06 — trpl c — trpl date — surgeon — OC — compl — eye — tr nr eye tot — op. time — rec — graft

07 — sut.rem date — failure date — end observ — date death — cause — M

CHECK UP DATES

date — clearness — cause — VA — ph/aph/pph — spher — cyl — direction — foto nr.

0. before trpl
1. after trpl

10
11
12
13
14
15
16

cell number is a link between the file which contains the serological data and phenotypes of the recipients and donors and the data base of the follow-up file. Data on the cause of death of the donor, the time interval between donor death and enucleation of the eye and between donor death and transplantation and storage methods were also recorded. The transplantation parameters covered by the follow-up forms are set out in table 1.

Table 1. Transplantation parameters

Diagn	-	diagnosis at transplant
PAD	-	histological diagnosis of the excised corneal button
Vasc.	-	degree of vascularisation of the recipient cornea
Bltr.	-	number of blood transfusions before the present transplantation
Preg.	-	number of pregnancies before the present transplantation
% LAL	-	lymphocyte antibody level before the present transplantation
vaccinations:		
Po	-	small pox
D	-	diphteria
K	-	whooping cough
T	-	tetanus
P	-	poliomyelitis
T	-	tropical diseases
O	-	others
inD	-	initial diagnosis
trpl. c	-	transplantation center
trpl. date	-	transplantation date
surgeon	-	name of the surgeon
OC	-	operation code lamellar/penetrating
compl	-	surgical complications
eye	-	eye operated
tr.nr. eye	-	number of transplantations on the eye considered
tr.nr. tot	-	total number of transplantations on both eyes
op time	-	duration of operation
O rec	-	diameter of the trephine used for the recipient
O graft	-	diameter of the trephine used for the donor button
sut.rem.date	-	suture removal date
failure date	-	failure date
end observ.	-	end observation
date death	-	death date of the recipient
cause	-	cause of graft failure
M	-	prospectively HLA matched +/-

In the first postoperative year, information on graft clarity, cause of decreased clarity (if present), visual acuity and refractive errors were recorded every 3 months. After the first year, these data were recorded every 6 months unless special events occurred, such as the major events like graft rejection, glaucoma and recurrence of the initial disease. All these data were stored on magnetic tape for eventual computer analysis. The necessity for subdividing the data according to various clinical criteria frequently reduced the number of cases within each subpopulations. Nevertheless, such analyses were performed and reported in order to present to other investigators the possibility for comparing their results with ours. The analytical techniques used for the follow-up analyses are set out in chapter 2. In chapter 5 the analysis of the different factors influencing corneal graft survival are described. Their effects were taken into account when analysing the effect of prospective HLA-A and -B matching on corneal allograft survival. This analysis is described in chapter 6.

During the period of this study (1976-1983), it became evident that the degree of matching for HLA-DR locus antigens was highly correlated with the level of kidney graft survival. In the eye HLA-DR locus antigens on dendritic cells (Langerhans cells) are located in the periphery of the cornea and along vascular structures (Mayer et al. 1983). Therefore, the interactions between HLA-DR, donor graft size and recipient cornea vascularisation on corneal graft survival were studied. The results are described in chapter 7.

Paediatric patients present their own special problems in corneal transplantation surgery. In cases of impaired visual acuity due to corneal opacities, the decision whether and when to perform a corneal transplantation is influenced not only by the corneal disease itself but also by the development of amblyopia, or worsening of the already existing amblyopia. The success of amblyopic treatment decreases with age. After 8 years of age increases in visual acuity by amblyopia training are seldom seen. In addition, the burden of a constantly inflamed eye as in recurrent herpes keratitis, which implies frequent visits to an ophthalmologist, constitutes a serious problem not only for the paediatric patients but also for their parents. Finally, if the corneal opacities are present on both eyes the normal development of the child may be severely affected. It is, therefore, evident that paediatric patients should be transplanted with a minimum of delay. The small number of successful grafts in very young children reported by several authors (Waring and Laibson 1977, Alberth 1980) prompted us to analyse the specific surgical and postoperative problems related to corneal transplantation in children. Special attention was given to infections, glaucoma, trauma, amblyopia and final visual outcome in this group of patients. The aim of this study was to obtain information which would help us to decide the optimal age for corneal transplantation in children (chapter 8).

In elderly patients, corneal endothelial decompensation following cataract extraction, whether or not combined with an intraocular lens insertion, is observed in a number of cases (Binkhorst, 1980). The most effective method of treatment is penetrating keratoplasty. The corneal graft survival of 136 patients with this diagnosis were analysed and described in chapter 9. The aim of the study was to investigate whether or not the presence of an intraocular lens influences corneal graft survival and consequently to establish indications for removing or retaining the lens at the time of graft surgery. We also investigated the effect of prospective HLA-A and -B matching on corneal graft survival in this subgroup of patients.

The recurrent character of herpes simplex virus keratitis leads to increasing scarring and opacity of the cornea. Imminent perforation or perforated descemetoceles are observed in severely inflamed corneas. The indication for corneal grafting in such patients is based not only on the possibilities for restoring the visual acuity but also the restoration of the integrity of the globe, or the elimination of the main part of the diseased cornea in the hope that the constant and invalidating recurrences of the herpes keratitis will disappear. Since the herpes simplex virus is a neurotropic virus, recurrences of herpes keratitis in the graft can be expected and are sometimes observed. Moreover the necessity of local dexamethason therapy after grafting can activate the herpes simplex virus. Especially in this group of patients the initial disease has an important influence on the final result of the corneal transplantation. The effect of prospective HLA-A and -B matching on corneal graft survival was studied in 288 patients with herpes simplex virus keratitis. The results were correlated with the recurrence of the herpes simplex infection (chapter 10).

Section III

Since 1976, cornea donors and recipients have been HLA typed with the purpose of obtaining the best possible match. The number of cases in the different diagnostic groups are now so large that it was possible to perform analyses of the distribution of the HLA and ABO antigens in different diagnostic groups as compared to those in a large group of normal individuals. The analyses of the HLA-A, -B and -C and ABO antigen frequencies in 114 patients with herpes simplex virus keratitis, 42 keratoconus patients, 23 patients with Fuchs' dystrophy and 44 patients with malignant choroidal melanoma are discribed in chapters 11, 13, 14 and 15 respectively. The HLA-DR antigen frequencies of 28 patients with herpes simplex virus keratitis were studied as well. The results are described in chapter 12.

References

Alberth B. (1980) Keratoplastik im Säuglings und Kindesalter. Klin. Mbl. Augenheilk. 177: 802-804.

Amos D.B. (1968) Human Histocompatibility locus HL-A. Science 159: 659.

Arentsen J.J., Morgan B. and Green W.R. (1976) Changing indication for keratoplasty. Am. J. Ophth. 81: 313-318.

Batchelor J.R., Casey T.A., Gibbs D.C., Lloyd D.F.,Werb A., Prasad S.S. and James A. (1976) HLA matching and corneal grafting. Lancet 1: 551-554.

Benacerraf B. (1981) Role of MHC gene products in immune regulation. Science 212: 1229.

Binkhorst C.D. (1980) Corneal and retinal complications after cataract extraction. Ophthalmol. 87, 7: 609-617.

Bloomfield S.E. (1980) Clinical allergy and immunology of the external eye. In Duane T.D. (ed). Clinical Ophthalmology 5, 28: 20-21.

Bodmer W.F. et al. (1966) Genetics of the '4' and 'LA' human leukocyte groups. Ann. N.J. Acad. Sci. 129 473.

Ceppelini R. et al. (1967) Genetics of leukocyte antigens. A family study of segregation and linkage. In: Histocompatibility Testing 1967, p. 149. Munksgaard, Copenhagen.

Ciba Foundation Symposium (1973) Corneal graft failure, p. 344. Associated Scientific Publishers, Amsterdam/London/New York.

Ciotola G. (1949) Considerazioni sulla cheratoplastica con particolare riguardo agli esiti tardivi. Bull. d'ocul. 28: 471-489.

Dausset J. (1954) Leuko-agglutinins. IV. Leuko-agglutinins and blood transfusion. Vox Sang. 4: 190.
Dausset J., Ivanyi P. and Ivanyi D. (1965) Tissue alloantigens in human: Identification of a complex system (HU-1) In: Histocompatibility Testing 1965, p. 51. Munksgaard, Copenhagen.
Dieffenbach J.F. (1831) Beitrage zur Verpflanzungder Hornhaut. Ztschr. f. d. Ophth. 1: 172-176.
Duquesnoy R.J., Marrari M. (1980) MB system. In: P.I. Terasaki, Ed. Histocompatibility Testing. Los Angeles, California. UCLA Tissue Typing Laboratory, 552–555.
Hensen E.J. (1983) An approach to study the genetic control of the antigen-specific immune response in man. Diss. Univ. of Leyden.
Jones B.R. (1973) Ciba Foundation Symposium; Corneal graft failure, p. 1. Associated Scientific Publishers, Amsterdam/London/New York.
Kissmeyer-Nielsen F., Svejgaard A. and Hange M. (1968) Genetics of the Human HL-A transplantation system. Nature 219: 1116.
Klein J., Juretic A., Baxevenis C.N. and Nagy Z.A. (1981) The traditional and a new version of the mouse H-2 complex. Nature 291: 455.
Löhnlein W. (1950) Über Keratoplastik. München med. Wohnsche. 92: 1201-1206.
Mayer D.J., Daar A.S., Casey T.A. and Fabre J.W.(1983). Localization of HLA-A, -B and -C and -DR antigens in the human cornea. Transplantation Proceedings vol. XV, no. 1: 126-129.
Medawar P.B. (1946) Immunity to homologous grafted skin II. The relationship between the antigens of blood and skin. Brit. J. Exp. Path. 27:15.
Miescher P. and Fauconnet M. (1954) Mise en evidence de differents groupes leucocytaires chez l'homme. Schweiz. Med. Wschr. 84: 597.
Nelken D. Histocompatibility antigens of the cornea.(1965) In: Histocompatibility Testing Munksgaard, Copenhagen.
Owens W.C., Frank J.J., Leahy B., Messier P.E., Scheie H.G., Vincent B.R., Wadsworth J.A.C. and Stansbury F.C. (1949) Results of corneal transplantations. Am. J. Ophth. 31: 1394-1399.
Payne R. and Rolfs M.R. (1958) Fetomaternal leukocyte incompatibility. J. Clin. Invest. 37: 1756.
Van Rood J.J., Eernisse J.G. and van Leeuwen A. (1958) Leukocyte antibodies in sera from pregnant women. Nature 181: 1735.
Van Rood J.J. (1962) Leukocyte grouping A method and its application. Thesis, University of Leiden.
Van Rood J.J. et al. (1965) Leukocyte groups, the normal lymphocyte transfer test and homograft sensitivity. In: Histocompatibility Testing 1965, p. 35. Munksgaard, Copenhagen.
Van Rood J.J., van Leeuwen A., Ploem J.S. (1976) Simultaneous detection of two cell population by two-colour fluorescence and application to recognition of B-cell determinants. Nature 262, 5571: 795.
Van Rood J.J. (1979) Microlymphocytotoxicity method. In: NIAID Manual of tissue typing techniques. (Ed: J. Ray) National Institute of Health (NIH) (80-545) Maryland, U.S.A., p. 104.
Roberts J.E. (1950) Statistics on results of keratoplasty. Am. J. Ophth. 33: (part 110) 21–23.
Sanfilippo F. (1982) Critical factors in corneal transplantation. SEOPF, 4.
Shaw S., Johnson A.H. and Shearer G.M. (1980) Evidence for a new segregant series of B cell antigens which are encoded in the HLA-D region and stimulate secondary allogeneic proliferative and cytotoxic responses. J. Exp. Med. 152: 565.
Smith R.E., McDonald R.H., Nesburn A.B. and Minckler D.S. (1980) Penetrating keratoplasty. Arch. Ophthalmol. 98: 1226-1229.
Spielman W. (1955) Serologische Grundlagen der Transfusionsstörungen. Bibli. Haemat. 2: 7.
Stansbury F.C. (1949) Corneal transplantations. Arch Ophth. 42: 813-844.
Terasaki P.I. and McClelland J.D. (1964) Microdroplet assay of human serum cytotoxins. Nature 204: 998.
Thomas C.J. (1955) The cornea, p. 1151. Charles C. Thomas Publishers, Springfield, Illinois, U.S.A.

De Vries R.R.P., Meerakhan P., Bernini L.F., van Loghem E., Van Rood J.J. (1979) Genetic control of survival in epidemies. J. Immunogenet 6: 271-287.
Waring G.O., Laibson P.R. (1977) Keratoplasty ininfants and children. Trans. Am. Acad. Ophthalmol. Otolaryngol. 83: 283-289.

CHAPTER 2

Statistical methods*

Introduction

Survival curves set out the probability for the occurrence of an event at particular points in time, i.e. graft function or patient survival. The two most commonly used methods for estimating actuarial survival curves are Life Table Estimates (Gehan, 1969) and Kaplan-Meier Product Limit Estimates (Kaplan and Meier, 1958). In both methods, patients may enter the study at different time intervals.

Life Table estimates utilize time intervals which are longer than the follow-up intervals. Follow-up intervals indicate the frequency with which graft function or patient survival are recorded, i.e. days, weeks, months, years, etc. In the Kaplan-Meier method, follow-up intervals are kept as short as possible, i.e. days. In both methods, survival estimates are calculated only for intervals in which events (graft failures or deaths) have occurred. A lucid comparison of the two methods has been reported by Sylvester et al. in 1978. The actuarial survival curves reported in this thesis have been computed within the Kaplan-Meier method (Kaplan and Meier, 1958), using the Follow-up Computer Program of the Department of Immunohaematology, Leyden University Hospital, and Eurotransplant.

Data-base

The data-base used for the follow-up analyses of corneal transplants is similar in structure to the one which is used for the follow-up analyses of renal transplants. Its records consist of personal, clinical and immunological data from the donor-recipient transplant pairs, dates of transplantation and of last follow-up and whether or not the graft is still functioning or, alternatively, the date of death of the recipient and numerous other parameters. The immunological data include the complete HLA phenotypes of the donor and recipient, the number of mismatched antigens in the HLA-A, -B, -C and -DR loci, whether or not the recipient has leukocyte

* *For colour plates, see pp. 72ff.*

antibodies etc. Parameters which are unique for corneal transplants, such as the diameter of the donor cornea button and the degree of vascularization of the host cornea, have been added to the records.

Method of computing life table estimates

The technique for calculating life tables is based upon the fact that 'beginning with time t=0 the probability of the graft surviving for (t+1) days after transplantation equals the probability of its surviving for t days, multiplied by the probability of neither rejection nor death on the next day. Gore (1984) and Breslow (1979) pointed out that it was 'because of this multiplicative structure, Kaplan and Meier refer to their estimate as the product limit (PL) estimate'. The above rather technical definition has been rephrased by Julian Peto (1983) using a minimum of statistical jargon. He states that 'the method of calculating the actuarial survival curve follows immediately from the observation that to survive a year a patient must survive the first day, and the second, an the third, and so on up to the 365th day. The separate probabilities of surviving each day are multiplied together, giving probability of surviving 365 days
= (Prob. for day 1) x (Prob. for day 2) x . . .
x (Prob. for days 364) x (Prob. for day 365).

Consider the following example:

Period	Cases	Functioning	Failed	Lost	%Func.	Cum.%
0	100	100	0	0	100.0	100.0
1	100	90	10	0	90.0	90.0
2	90	70	20	0	77.8	70.0
3	70	70	0	0	100.0	70.0
4	70	55(60)	5	10	92.3	64.6

Period 0 presents no analytical problems. It represents the beginning of the study. Consequently, all cases (grafts) are still functioning and %Func. and Cum.% (Cummulative % or Actuarial %) are both 100%.

In period 1, 90 grafts were still functioning, 10 have failed and 0 cases were lost to observation. The proportion of functioning grafts equals the number of functioning grafts divided by the number of cases at risk (the sum of the number of functioning and the number of failed grafts), i.e. 90/100 = 0.900 = 90.0% = %Func. The cumulative (actuarial) percentage equals the %Func. for this period multiplied by the Cum.% at the end of the previous period, i.e. 90.0% x 100.0% = 90.0%.

In period 2, 70 of the 90 grafts which were still functioning in period 1 are still functioning, 20 failed and 0 cases were lost to observation. The proportion of functioning grafts (%Func.) equals 70/90 = 0.778 = 77.8% =

%Func. The cumulative (actuarial) percentage equals the %Func. for this period multiplied by the Cum.% at the end of the previous period, i.e. 77.8% x 90.0% = 70.0%.

There have been no failures in period 3, therefore %Func. = 100.0. Consequently, there is no change in Cum.%. This example illustrates the fact that calculations need to be carried out only for periods in which failures have occurred.

Period 4 contains 10 cases which have been lost to observation. Consequently, it cannot be determined whether or not those grafts are still functioning. The most probable reasons for those losses are that the graft recipients have changed their addresses or that they have emigrated to another country without notifying their transplantation or follow-up centers.

Because of these 10 losses, there is some degree of uncertainty with regard to the number of cases at risk in period 4, i.e. the number of cases which could have been exposed to the risk of failing in this period. Julian Peto suggests that it will be on average less than the 'number functioning in the previous period and greater than this number minus the number lost since the last follow-up period, hence a reasonable approximation is to average these numbers' (Peto, 1983). That suggestion has been followed by adding 1/2 of the losses to the number functioning in the period 4. The number of functioning cases has been increased from 55 to 55 + (1/2 of 10) = 60 and that value has been used for the calculation of %Func. and Cum.%. The proportion of functioning grafts equals 60/65 = 0.923 = 92.3% = %Func. The cumulative (actuarial) percentage equals the %Func. for this period multiplied by the Cum.% at the end of the previous period, i.e. 92.3% x 70.0% = 64.6%.

Actuarial survival curves are displayed on arithmetic graph paper, with the probability of survival on the y axis and follow-up time on the x axis. The technique illustrated in the above example apply also when multiple curves are to be displayed on the same plot. When multiple curves are displayed, a unique character, usually the curve number, is used for the different curves. The meanings of the identity characters are indicated in a legend at the upper right of the plot. The calculations for one curve are not influenced by the calculations for any other curves.

Standard error of life table estimates

The standard errors (S.E.) of the life table estimates, for example, graft function (Cum.%), are calculated with the following formula:

$$\text{S.E.} = \text{Cum.\%} \times \sqrt{(1 - \text{Cum.\%}) / N},$$

where N = number of grafts still functioning. The standard error indicates the degree of variability in this life table estimate.

The 95% confidence limits of the life table table estimates of graft function at a particular time are equal to: Cum.% +/- (1.96 x S.E.).

Note that the magnitude of the standard error is inversely proportional to N, consequently, small numbers of cases at risk in a period generate wide confidence limits.

Significance testing, the logrank test

Comparisons of two or more survival curves are usually made with a statistical procedure first proposed by Mantel in 1966 and named the Longrank Testby R. Peto et al. in 1976 and 1977. The test is based upon the premise that, if there are no differences in the effects of two or more treatments the number of events (graft failures, deaths, etc.) in each treatment class should be in the same proportion to the numbers of cases (patients) in the different classes. For example: if there are 100, 200 and 300 patients in classes I, II and III respectively, and a total of 60 events (deaths) are observed, then we would expect 60 x (100/600) = 10 deaths in class I, 60 x (200/600) = 20 deaths in class II and 60 x (300/600) = 30 deaths in class III. For the sake of simplicity, we will use the term 'Expectations' instead of the phrase 'Extent of exposure to risk of death (failure)' which is used in the formal description of the Logrank test.

The significance of the differences between the numbers of Observed(O) and Expected(E) events is assessed by means of a chi square statistic based upon the sum of the $(O-E)^2/E$ values from all the classes. The number of degrees of freedom is equal to the number of classes minus 1, i.e. in the above example it equals 3 - 1 = 2. Consider the following example(table 1): the data

Table 1. Data and intermediate values for the Logrank Test

	Small			Medium			Large		
		Failures			Failures			Failures	
Period	Func.	Obs.	Exp.	Func.	Obs.	Exp.	Func.	Obs.	Exp.
0	194.8			338.0			289.0		
1	188.5	4	7.6	324.5	11	13.2	270.0	17	11.3
2	182.0	3	5.5	312.0	7	9.5	255.0	13	8.0
3	175.5	1	2.9	302.5	2	5.0	245.0	9	4.1
4	166.0	2	4.1	288.5	6	7.1	232.5	9	5.8
5	159.0	2	1.7	282.5	1	2.9	226.0	4	2.4
6	152.0	2	1.9	278.5	1	3.4	220.5	5	2.7
9	136.5	3	7.2	254.5	13	13.8	199.5	16	11.1
12	121.5	4	5.5	219.5	7	10.0	181.0	13	8.5
18	105.5	2	4.9	191.0	11	9.2	163.5	9	7.9
24	84.0	2	4.1	150.5	7	7.6	141.5	10	7.3
36	33.5	9	4.8	65.5	5	8.0	65.0	7	8.2
Totals		34	50.1		71	89.6		112	77.3

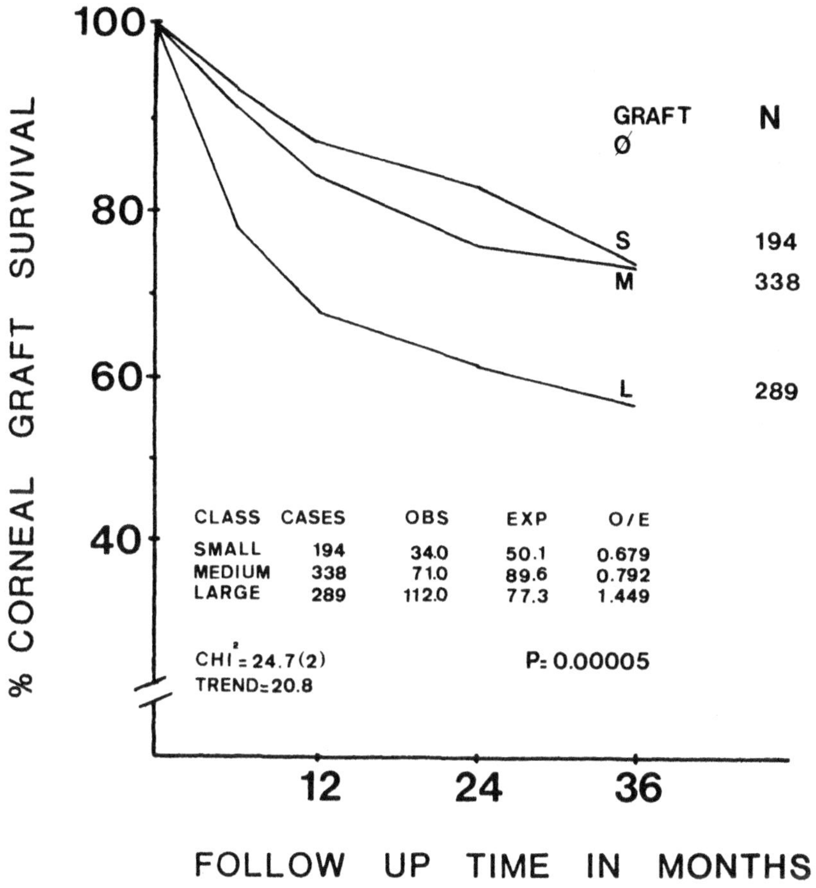

Figure 1. The effect of graft diameter on corneal graft survival (N=821).

are presented in figure 1A which is copied from chapter 7.

Using the data from period 2 in this table, the calculation of the expected numbers of failures in the 3 classes will be described. The numbers of cases are 182 + 3 = 185, 312 + 7 = 319 and 255 + 13 = 268 in the 3 classes respectively, with a grand total of 772. The calculations for the numbers of expected failures proceeds as shown in table 2.

Table 2. Calculation of Expected Failures

Class	Cases	Expected Failures
Small	185	185 / 772 × 23 = 5.5
Medium	319	319 / 772 × 23 = 9.5
Large	268	268 / 772 × 23 = 8.0

After the calculations of the numbers of expected failures in the 3 classes have been carried out over all of the periods, the significance of the differences between the 3 classes is determined. For that purpose the class totals which are indicated at the bottom of table 1 are used. A summary of the results of the Logrank Test are presented in table 3.

Table 3. Summary of the Logrank Test for the differential effect of cornea donor button size and corneal graft function

Class	Cases	Obs.	Exp.	O/E	$(O-E)^2/E$
Small	194	34.0	50.1	0.679	5.2
Medium	338	71.0	89.6	0.792	3.9
Large	289	112.0	77.3	1.449	15.6

Chi square for heterogeneity = 24.7 (2 degrees of freedom) $p = 0.0005$

When three or more classes can be logically ranked into a natural order in a non-arbitrary way, such as Small, Medium and Large or 0, 1 and 2 HLA-DR mismatches, it is important to determine if there is a statistically significant tendency for a trend in prognosis as we go from Class 1 to Class 2 to Class 3 (Peto et al. 1977). Using the technique described by those same authors, the calculation proceeds as shown in table 4.

Table 4. Test for Trend

n	Class	Obs.	Exp.	$(O-E)^2/E$	A	B	C
1	Small	34.0	50.1	5.2	-16.1	50.1	50.1
2	Medium	71.0	89.6	3.9	-37.2	179.2	358.4
3	Large	112.0	77.3	15.6	104.1	231.9	695.7
Totals		217.0	217.0	24.7	50.8	461.2	1104.2
Total names		Osum	Esum	X^2	Asum	Bsum	Csum

Chi square for trend = 20.8 (1 degree of freedom) $p = 0.00006$
n = class number
$A = n \times (O-E)$
$B = n \times E$
$C = n \times n \times E$
$V = Csum-(Bsum \times Bsum/Esum)$
chi square = $Asum \times Asum/V$

General remarks

Since the Logrank Test assesses the significance of differences between the numbers of Observed and Expected events, i.e. failures, deaths, etc; the number of cases at the beginning of a study should be large enough so that the number of events observed in the different classes will be large enough to provide a reasonable chance of detecting a significant difference between the classes. In simpler terms, the number of events is more critical than the number of cases.

Since the onset of rejection of allografts is, in general not a very rapid procedure it is improper to consider the differences between two survival curves at a single point in time rather than their overall differences.

When inspecting reports which contain summaries of Logrank analyses, it is useful to examine the relationships between the O/E ratios in the different classes (Peto et al. 1977). The O/E ratios represent the relative failure rates in a particular class. A cursory examination of the summary which is set out in table 3 reveals that the difference between the ratios for the Small and Medium classes (0.113) is small compared to the difference between these two individual classes and the Large class (0.770 and 0.657 respectively). The ratio of the O/E values for Small/Large (0.679 / 1.449 = 0.469) suggests that the true failure rate ratio is 0.469, i.e. that the use of Small donor cornea buttons prevents or delays about 53% (1 - 0.469 = 0.531) of corneal graft failures. In a similar manner, a comparison of the O/E values for Medium/Large (0.792 / 1.449 = 0.547) suggests that the use of Medium sized donor cornea buttons may prevent or delay about 45% (1 - 0.547 = 0.453) of corneal graft failures. The results of those comparisons may provide useful information to clinicians, even in the absence of statistical significance, especially when relatively few failures have been observed.

When performing analyses which generate large numbers of comparisons, the chance of observing random deviations, with significant p values, may become large. In the numerous studies of the differential frequencies of the HLA antigens in patients and in healthy controls, p values are frequently corrected for the total number of comparisons which have been made, using either Weiner's method (Weiner 1970) which is an overcorrection or Edward's method (Edwards 1974). That practice is not followed for the results of survival studies. Nevertheless, the risk of making Type I decision errors, with rejection of the null hypothesis for no significant difference between two classes, may be ignored because the results of such studies are considered as provisional, pending confirmation by similar studies in other centers.

References

Breslow N.E. (1979) Statistical methods for censored survival data. Environmental Health Perspectives, 32: 181-192.

Edwards J.U. (1974) HLA and disease. The detection of associations. J. Immunogenet. 1: 249-256.

Gehan E.A. (1969) Estimating survival functions from the life table method. J.Chron.Dis. 21: 629-635.

Gore S.M. (1984) Graft survival after renal transplantation: agenda for analysis. Kidney International. in press.

Kaplan E.L. and Meier P. (1958) Non parametric estimation from incomplete observations. JAMA 53: 457.
Mantel N. (1966) Evaluation of survival data and two new rank order statistics arising in its consideration. Cancer Chemother. Rep. 50: 163.
Peto J. (1984) The calculation and interpretation of survival curves. Oxford University Press. In press.
Peto R., Pike M.C., Armitage P., Breslow N.E., Cox D.R., Howard S.V., Mantel N., McPherson K., Peto J. and Smith P.G. (1976) Design and analysis of randomized clinical trials requiring prolonged observation of each patient. Part I, Introduction and design J. Cancer 34: 585-612.
Peto R., Pike M.C., Armitage P., Breslow N.E., Cox D.R., Howard S.V., Mantel N., McPherson K., Peto J. and Smith P.G. (1977) Design and analysis of randomized clinical trials requiring prolonged observation of each patient. Part II, Analysis and examples J. Cancer 35: 1-39.
Sylvester R.J., Mackin D. and Staquet M.J. (1978) A comparison of the alternative methods of calculating survival curves arising from clinical trials. Biomedicine Special Issue 28: 49-53.
Weiner A.S. (1970) Blood groups and disease. Am.J.Hum. Genet. 22: 476-483.

SECTION I

Donor corneas from eyes containing a malignant choroidal melanoma

CHAPTER 3

Longterm follow-up study of 19 patients who received 22 corneal grafts between 1939 and 1948 from eyes enucleated because of malignant choroidal melanoma*

Summary

A longterm follow-up study of 19 patients who received 22 corneal grafts between 1939 and 1948 from eyes containing a malignant choroidal melanoma revealed no evidence for the transmission of tumour cells by corneal transplantation. A negative effect on the life expectancies of the recipients of this donor material could not be established, nevertheless the use of such corneal grafts is not advised because of poorer graft survival when compared to the survival of grafts from other sources.

Introduction

In 1934, Filatov published the first report on the use of cadaveric donor material for corneal transplantation. Before that time, the only source of donor corneas were eyes enucleated for serious ailments, but with transparant corneas. However, that did not happen very often. In The Netherlands, corneal grafting was started in 1939 in the University Eye Clinic, Leyden. Up to 1946, the ophthalmologists did not dare to use cadaveric donor material because they did not trust the quality of the donor cornea. After september 1946,they started to use not only corneas from eyes enucleated because of intraocular tumours but also corneas from deceased individuals. Since no studies have been reported on the longterm consequences of using donor cornea material from eyes enucleated because of intraocular tumours, we decided to do so. To that end, we will report the results of a longterm follow-up study of corneal transplantations performed with donor corneas obtained from eyes which were enucleated because of malignant choroidal melanoma (M.C.M.).

All survival times were calculated using the actuarial life table method. The significance of the differences between the various classes were tested with X^2 statistics derived from the log rank test (Peto et al. 1976). The numbers to the right of the follow-up curve (see fig. 3) indicate the number of patients at risk at the start of the study.

* *For colour plates, see pp. 72ff.*

Methods and material

From June 1939 until December 1948, 22 penetrating corneal transplantations were performed with donor corneas from eyes enucleated because of an intraocular tumour. At that time if possible, two squared grafts from one donor cornea were prepared (fig. 1). Thirteen enucleated eyes were used. From nine corneas double grafts were prepared and from the remaining four, single grafts were prepared. The histological reports of these 13 eyes revealed that they were all enucleated due to the presence of a malignant choroidal melanoma. The histological description of the tumours was most alarming. Only a single case consisted of a small posterior pole tumour without scleral ingrowth. Scleral perforation or ingrowth in the sclera by the tumour was recorded in 6 cases, one of which is presented in fig. 2, while extension into the vitreous was recorded in 5 cases. Two tumours originated in the ciliary body. These corneas were used for 4 transplantations. Tumour diameters were not measured at that time but they were classified as 'very large' in 9 cases. In two of them it was noted that those tumours filled approximately one half and the entire vitreous cavity respectively. A description of the histological cell types of the tumours was made only in the last three cases; one tumour contained spindle cells only while the other two were composed of epitheloid cells with a few spindle cells. All donor corneas

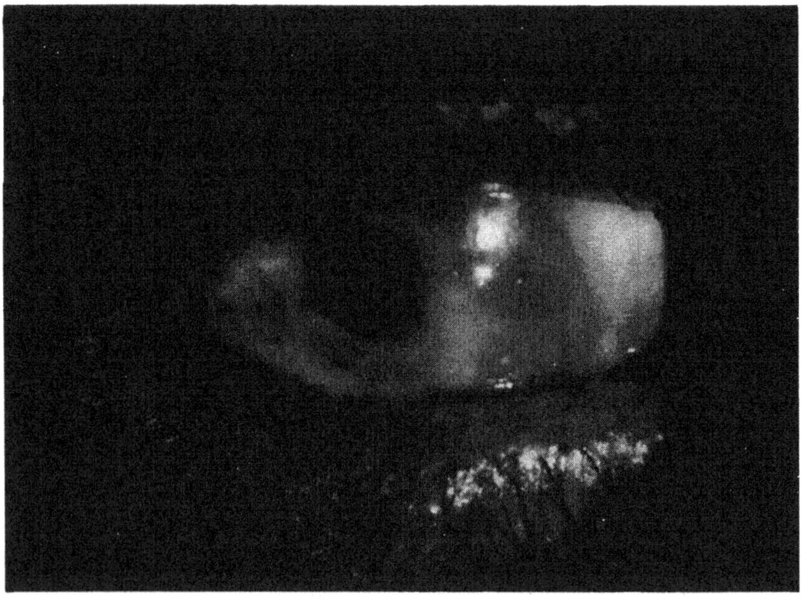

Figure 1. Squared corneal graft, performed in September 1939 in a 27 years old patient. The graft is still functioning, visual acuity is 0.3 after correction.

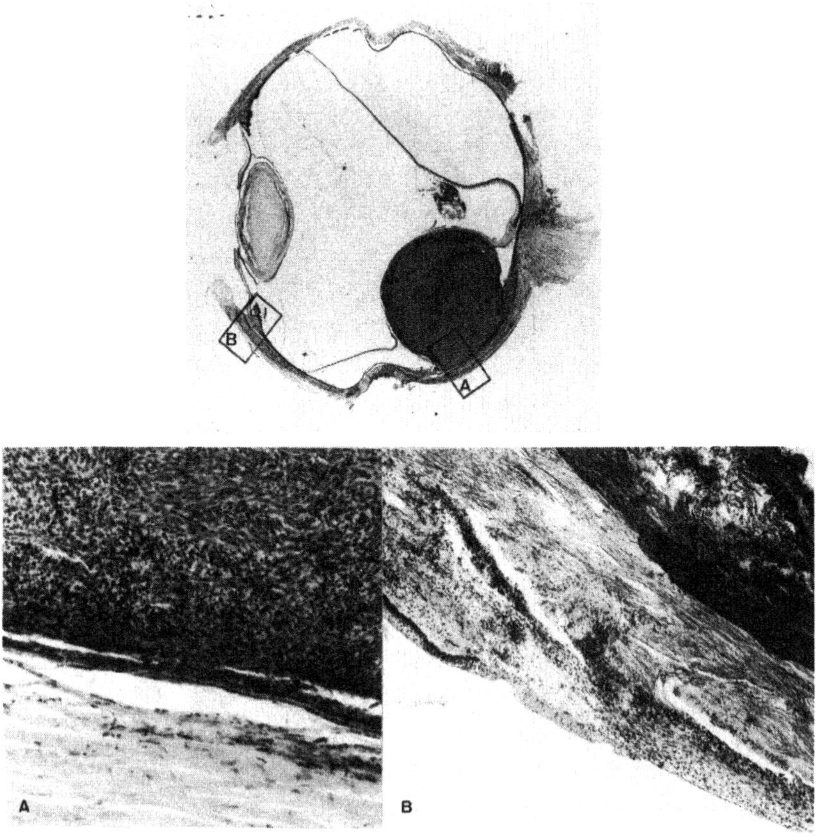

Figure 2. Bulbus enucleated in 1946 containing a malignant choroidal melanoma, with scleral ingrowth by the tumour (A) and protusion into the vitreous. The central part of the cornea is excised and used for corneal transplantation. Note the subepithelial lymphocytic infiltration close to the excised corneal part. (B) (with the courtesy of prof J.A. Oosterhuis)

were used within 24 hours after enucleation, and, if necessary, stored in a moist chamber at 4 °C.

The 19 recipients (8 female, 11 male), 3 of whom were grafted for a second time with this type of donor material, varied in age at the time of transplatation from 10 to 65 years. Only 3 of these 19 patients are still under regular ophthalmological supervision by one of the authors (Kok-van Alphen). The remaining 16 were traced with the help of the registrar offices in their last known places of residence. Twelve patients died between 1944 and 1982. Information on the four living patients followed-up elsewhere was obtained either from their ophthalmologists and / or their family doctors. For deceased patients, information was obtained from the registrar's office in each municipality where the patient resided and information about the cause of death, as indicated on the death certificates was obtained from the offices of vital statistics with the help of the National Public Health Service. The family doctors and/or the physicians who signed the death certificates were interviewed personally by one of us. Special attention was paid to information on the general health of the patients during their last years and to the occurrence of malignancies. If available, information about the histology of the malignancies was obtained. From 1948 onwards, malignant melanoma was assigned a specific code number by the offices of vital statistics.

Results

The ophthalmologic diagnoses at the time of transplantation of the 19 patients who received 22 grafts from donor eyes containing a M.C.M., are summarised in table 1. The follow-up period was 3 to 44 years, average 28.6 years.

The survival of the corneal allografts in those 22 transplantations performed between 1939 and 1948 was poor (curve I fig. 3). For comparison curve II represents the corneal allograft survival of 44 patients grafted between 1976 and 1981 with donor corneas also from eyes containing a M.C.M. The significant difference (overall $p=0.00065$) in graft survival is the result of four decades of technical improvements in corneal graft surgery.

Twelve of the 19 patients who received a corneal graft between 1939 and 1948 died between 3 and 34 years after transplantation. Their causes of death are listed in table 2. Two patients died because of a malignancy, 9 and 17 years after the corneal transplantation. A histological description of the tumour was available, a fibrosarcoma in one case and an adenocarcinoma in the other case. One patient who died 34 years after corneal transplantation because of cardiac decompensation was suspected to have a gastro-intestinal

Table 1. Ophthalmic diagnosis at transplantation of 22 corneas grafted between 1939 and 1948

Diagnosis	Number of cases
Parenchymatosis	5
Scrophulosis	3
Groenow's degeneration	3
Inflammation	2
Keratitis eci	2
Herpes simplex keratitis	1
Chemical burns	1
Acne rosacea keratitis	1
Pemphigus	1
Lipoidosis	1
Failure of a previous graft	2

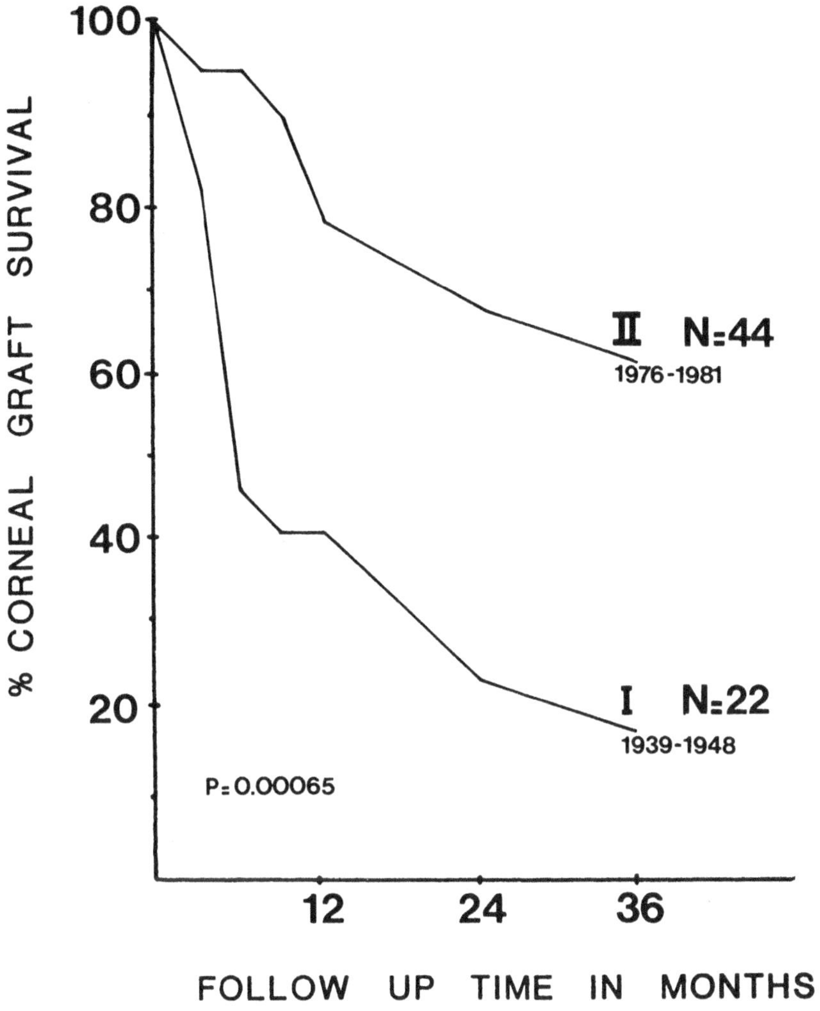

Figure 3. Survival of corneal allografts from donors with malignant choroidal melanoma in the different time periods.

malignancy as well. Extensive diagnostic investigations were not carried out on this 78 year old woman and postmortem examination was refused by her family.

The ages of the patients at the time of corneal transplantation, their subsequent survival (in years) and their life expectancies (Source: 'Centraal Bureau voor de Statistiek', 1975) are set out in fig. 4. The ages at the time of transplantation of the twelve patients who later died ranged from 37 to 65 years and their survival after transplantation ranged from 3 to 34 years, average 21.5 years.

Table 2. Cause of death (according to death certificates) of 12 transplant recipients grafted between 1939 and 1948

Cause of death	Number of cases
Cardiac decompensation	3
Heart attack	3
Arterial insufficiency	1
Accident	1
Cerebrovascular accident	1
Tuberculosis	1
Fibrosarcoma of liver and gal bladder	1
Adenocarcinoma of the pancreas	1

Discussion

The possibility of the transfer of malignant melanoma cells to the recipient as the result of using corneas from eyes with a M.C.M. should be seriously considered. Clinical manifestations of such transfers may not be limited to the growth of an intraocular tumour in the grafted eye. Haematogenous dissemination of malignant melanoma cells is a common cause of metastasis of these tumours (Einhorn et al. 1974). Manschot and

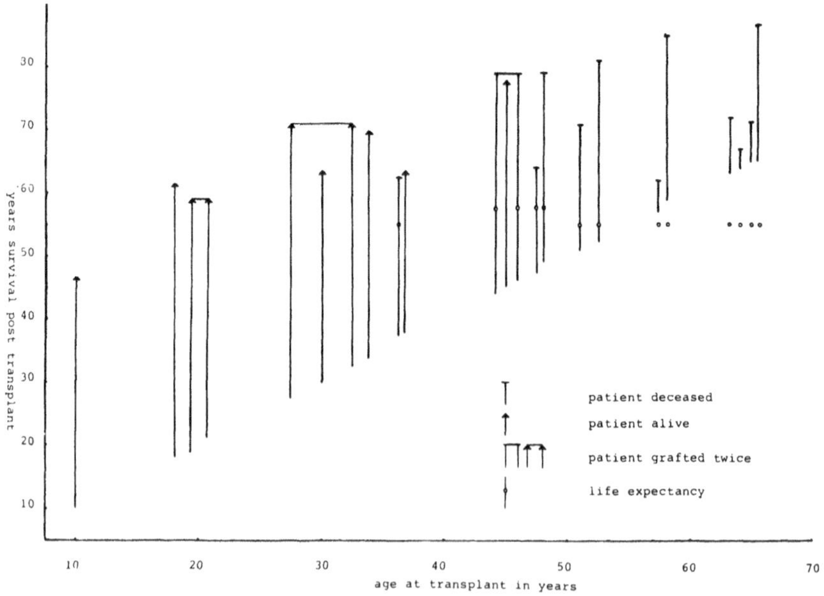

Figure 4. Age at transplant and survival post transplant versus life expectancy of 19 patients who received 22 corneal grafts between 1939 and 1948 from eyes enucleated because of malignant choroidal melanoma.

Van Peperzeel (1980) applied the growth curve for a hypothetical tumour from Collins et al. (1956) to malignant choroidal melanomas. In this way they calculated the maximum possible variation in interval between the time of enucleation of an eye containing a M.C.M. and the detection of metastasis as 0.6 to 8.2 years for the epitheloid cell type melanoma and 2 to 28 years for the spindle cell type melanoma. Jensen (1982) reported on a patient in whom metastasis appeared 23 years after enucleation. Consequently, the confirmation of a possible recurrence requires follow-up periods clearly in excess of 28 years. In the material we analysed the last corneal graft was performed in 1948, 35 years ago. We found no intra- ocular tumours and none of the patients died from a malignant melanoma. The life expectancies of the patients did not seem to be adversely affected due to the use of corneas from eyes enucleated because of M.C.M. The death of two patients who died with a systemic malignancy was clearly not due to metastases of the M.C.M.

Zakov et al. (1978) advised that: 'extreme caution should be used in selecting eyes of patients with ocular or systemic malignancy'. The possibility of transmission of oncogenic virus particles led this author to suggest that every patient dying of a systemic malignancy should be rejected as a source of donor material. Biochemical findings in favour of a viral etiology of human cancer are the demonstration of viral specific RNA in human breast carcinomas (Spiegelmann et al. 1972), leukemias (Baxt and Spiegelmann 1972) and lymphomas (Hehlman et al. 1972). Demonstration of a viral etiology for melanomas in hamsters was unsuccessful (Birkmayer et al. 1974), although cell-free transmission of the tumour has been reported (Epstein et al. 1968). The longterm follow-up of 22 corneal grafts from enucleated eyes containing a malignant choroidal melanoma is an additional argument against the possible transmission aetiology of these tumours through a viral agent.

Cassen et al. (1983) reported the presence of neoplastic cells situated paracentrally in the cornea of a patient who died of acute myelogenous leukemia; the choroid was massively infiltrated with leukemic blastcells. However, no information on the eventual occurrence of leukemia in the recipient was possible.

Conclusions

Despite the large malignant melanomas described in the histological reports of the enucleated eyes used for 22 corneal grafts in this study, the limited tools for investigation of the donor eyes before grafting in the period 1939-1948 and the longterm follow-up periods, we did not observe any evidence for the transmission of malignant choroidal melanomas. Nevertheless, we do not advise the use of such donors since further studies (chapter 4) revealed that such grafts have a poorer survival than grafts from other sources.

Acknowledgements

We thank prof. Dr. J.A. Oosterhuis for allowing to publish these cases from the Leyden University Hospital.

Thanks to the well kept ophthalmological archives we were able to trace the case histories of all the patients and the histological descriptions of all the donor eyes in this study. The late Mr. L. Beumer and Mr. P. de Sera have been of great help in this respect. Mr. J. van Delft and Mr. E. Barthen were very helpful with the search for old histological preparations. Dr. J.J.P. Pieters of the National Public Health Service and Dr. L.M. Friden-Kill of the Bureau of Vital Statistics have been of great help in finding the causes of death of the deceased patients.

References

Baxt W.G. and Spiegelman S. (1972) Nuclear DNA sequences present in human leukemic cells and absent normal leucocytes. Proc. Nat. Acad. Sci U.S.A. 69: 3737.

Birkmayer G.D., Balda B.R. and Miller F. (1974) Onco-viral information in human melanoma. Europ. J. Cancer 10: 419.

Cassen J.H., Meisler D.M., Zakov Z.M. and Langston R.H.S. (1983) Donor material for corneal grafting. Am.J.Ophthalmol. 95, no. 5: 711-712.

Centraal Bureau v.d. Statistiek (1975) 75 Jaar statistiek in Nederland. Staatsuitgeverij, Den Haag, p. 19.

Collins V.P., Loeffler R.D. and Tivey H. (1956) Observation on growth rates of human tumors. Am.J.Roentgenol. 76: 989.

Einhorn L., Burgers M. and Gottlieb J. (1974) Metastatic patterns of choroidal melanoma. Cancer 34: 1001.

Epstein W.R., Fukuyama K., Benn M., Keston A.S. and Brandt R.B. (1968) Transmission of a pigmented melanoma in golden hamster by a cell-free ultra filtrats. Nature (London) 219: 979.

Filatov V.P. (1934) The cadaver's cornea for corneal transplantation. Sovet Vestnik Oftal. 4: 223.

Hehlman R., Kufe D. and Spiegelman S. (1972) Viral related RNA in Hodgkin's disease and other lymphomas. Proc. Nat. Acad. Sci. U.S.A. 69: 1729.

Jensen O.A. (1982) Malignant melanomas of the human uvea, 25 years follow-up in cases in Denmark, 1943-1952. Acta Ophthalmol. 60: 161.

Manschot W.A. and Peperzeel van H.A. (1980) Choroidal melanoma; enucleation or observation? A new approach. Arch. Ophthalmol. 98: 71.

Spiegelman S., Axel R. and Sehlom J. (1972) Virus related RNA in human and mouse mammary tumors. J.Nat. Cancer Inst. 48: 1205.

Zakov Z.N., Dohlman C.H., Perry H.D. and Albert D.M. (1978) Corneal donor material selection. Am.J.Ophthalmol. 86: 605.

CHAPTER 4

Survival of 44 corneal grafts obtained from eyes enucleated because of malignant choroidal melanoma*

Summary

Análysis of the survival of corneal grafts obtained from eyes enucleated because of malignant choroidal melanoma and of grafts from donors deceased of systemic malignancies revealed a large excess of graft failures in the malignant choroidal melanoma groups (O/E=1.454) as compared to the systemic malignancies group (O/E=0.857). When only HLA-A and -B well matched donor-recipient pairs in both groups were studied again a large excess of graft failures was observed in the malignant choroidal melanoma group (O/E=1.381) as compared to the systemic malignancies group (O/E=0.564).

The poor graft survival of grafts obtained from eyes enucleated because of malignant choroidal melanoma was due to an increased number of irreversible rejections. This number was significantly different from the number of irreversible rejections observed in grafts from donors deceased of systemic malignancies ($p=0.03$).

Introduction

In chapter 5 we show that the cause of death of a corneal donor did not significantly influence corneal graft survival. The aim of this study was to investigate whether there was a significant difference in the survival of corneal grafts obtained from eyes enucleated because of malignant choroidal melanoma and grafts obtained from donors who died because of systemic malignancies.

Materials and methods

Between January 1976 and January 1983 the causes of death of 590 corneal donors were recorded in the following categories: road traffic accident, cerebrovascular accident, cardiac failure, carcinoma and miscellaneous. The 'cause of death' was recorded as a carcinoma for 44 eyes previously enucleated because of a malignant choroidal melanoma (M.C.M.). Furthermore, information on sex and age of the donor, time interval between death and enucleation and time interval between death and transplantation were recorded. For eyes enucleated because of M.C.M. the

* *For colour plates, see pp. 72ff.*

time interval between 'death' and enucleation was recorded as zero while the time interval between 'death' and transplantation was measured from the moment that enucleation was performed and the time of transplantation.

Corneal donor material was either stored in McCarey Kaufman tissue culture medium or taken directly from the globe and stored in a moist chamber at +4 ° C, in this second instance it was always used within 24 hours. After the decision was made by others that enucleation of an eye with the clinical diagnosis of malignant choroidal melanoma was inevitable we examined the eye in order to decide if the cornea was suitable for transplantation. The cornea was used on condition that the tumour was restricted to the posterior pole of the eye and that the margins of the tumour were clearly defined. Protusion of the tumour of more than 3 diopters and/or the presence of one or more pigmented cells in the vitreous were contraindications. After the cornea had been removed histological examination of the globe was performed in order to confirm the clinical diagnosis of M.C.M.

All keratoplasties were performed by one of two surgeons (Völker-Dieben and Kok-van Alphen). Their surgical techniques were identical and were similar to the method described by Harms and Mackensen (1966). Postoperative care was not changed during the period of this study and has been previously described (Völker-Dieben et al. 1982).

HLA-A and -B typings were performed on all of the 44 donors with M.C.M. but only on 47 of the 158 donors with a systemic malignancy. HLA matching of donor and recipients was restricted to high risk patients: i.e. those with vascularised corneas and those with previous corneal graft rejections (chapter 6). If no suitable high risk recipient was available, because of more than two mismatches, the donor cornea was used randomly for a non-high risk patient. Five of the 47 typed corneas from donors who died from a systemic malignancy and four of the 44 corneas obtained from enucleated eyes because of M.C.M. were used randomly for a non-high risk patient. All HLA typings of patients and donors were performed with a standard microlymphocytotoxicity assay (Van Rood 1979) in the National Reference Center in Leiden (Department of Immunohaematology, University Hospital) with a serum set which recognises all official HLA and workshop specificities.

All patients and graft donors were of Dutch Caucasoid origin. Survival times were calculated using the actuarial life table method. The significance of the differences between the various classes were tested with X^2 derived from the logrank test (Peto et al. 1976). The numbers to the right of the follow-up curves (fig. 1-3) indicate the number of patients at risk at the start of the study.

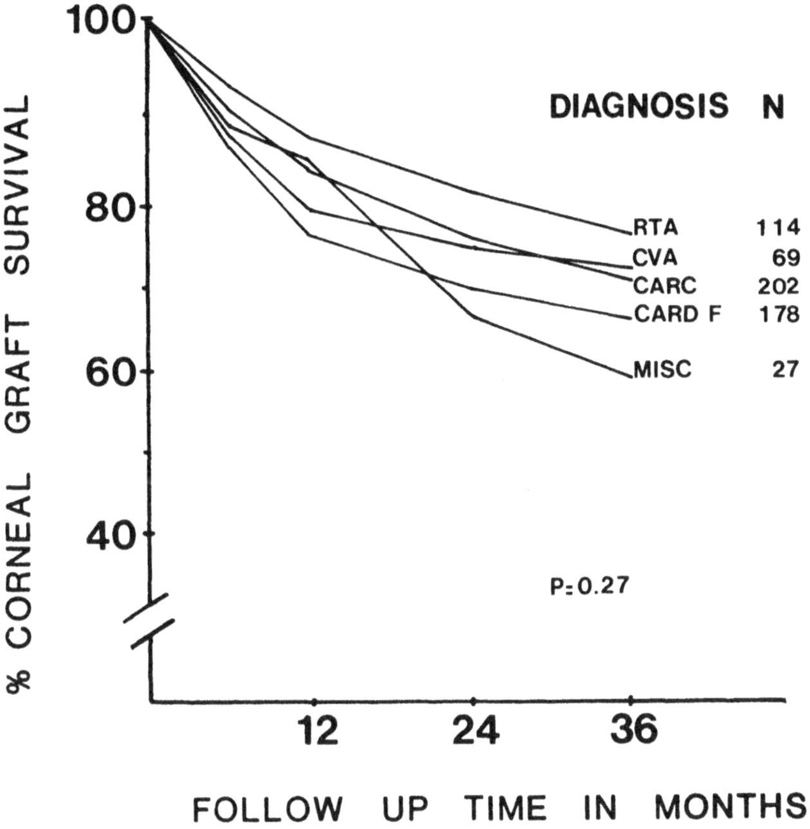

Figure 1. Relation between cause of death of the donor. RTA = road traffic accident; CVA = cerebro vascular accident; CARC = carcinoma; CARD F = cardiac failure; MISC = miscellaneous.

Results

Fig. 1 shows the graft survival per year for all patients transplanted since 1976. It can be seen that the one year graft survival improved from 71.5% in 1976 to 85.7% in 1978 and was followed by a decrease to 75.6% in 1979 and that it was 96% in 1980, the time of this publication.

Considering all 539 grafts fig. 2 shows a significant influence of previous graft failures on the graft outcome ($p<0.004$). The survival of first grafts at 12 months was 83.4% versus second and subsequent graft survival 74.6% or less.

Another highly significant influence was found in the degree of vascularisation of the host cornea ($p<0.00001$). Fig. 3 shows a one year graft survival of 100 and 91.4% respectively in none or slightly vascularized host corneas versus 70 and 69.5% in moderate or severely vascularized corneas.

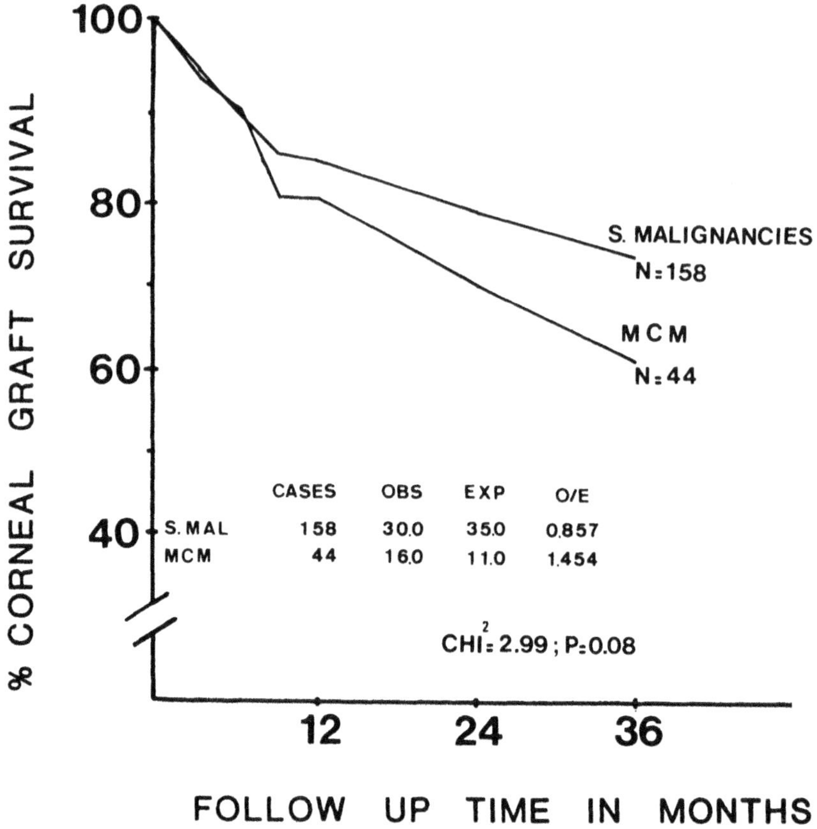

Figure 2. Analysis of survival of corneal grafts from donors deceased of systemic malignancies (S.MAL) and from eyes enucleated because of a malignant choroidal melanoma (MCM).

Negative influences on corneal graft survival are reported to be associated with: previous graft failure, vascularisation of the recipient cornea and large corneal graft diameter; while a positive influence was observed when grafts from female donors were transplanted into female recipients as compared to male recipients (chapter 5). The significantly better graft survival of HLA-A and -B matched grafts as compared to unmatched grafts in vascularised corneas, independent of the initial diagnosis at the time of transplantation, is reported in chapter 6. This observation was confirmed in 1983 in a selected group of herpes keratitis patients (chapter 11).

Table 1 compares both in number of patients and in percentages the distribution of factors which influence corneal graft survival in the group of donor eyes from patients with systemic malignancies with those from eyes enucleated because of M.C.M. Only the levels of HLA-A and -B matching in the two groups were significantly different uncorrected for the

Table 1. Factors influencing corneal graft survival

	Grafts from donors deceased of systemic malignancies (N=158)		Grafts from eyes enucleated because of M.C.M. (N=44)	
NEGATIVE				
- previous graft failures	58	(36.7%)	25	(56.8%)
- vascularised recipients	100	(63.2%)	37	(84.0%)
- large corneal graft diameter	54	(34.1%)	17	(38.6%)
POSITIVE				
- female donor - female recipient combination	37	(23.4%)	6	(13.6%)
- HLA-A and -B matching	42*	(26.5%)	40*	(90.9%)

* Degree of HLA-A and -B matching was significantly different $X^2 = 56.42$, uncorrected $p = 0.0005$

multiple comparisons which have been made (X^2=56.42, p=0.0005). Note that although the proportion of individuals well matched for HLA-A and -B was 90.9% in donor-recipient combinations wherein the donor corneas were obtained from eyes enucleated because of M.C.M., the survival of those grafts was inferior (fig. 2) to that of those in the other class where only 26.5% of the pairs were well matched for HLA-A and -B. Since it was unlikely that the high level of HLA-A and -B matching was the reason for the poor survival of M.C.M. grafts, we decided to repeat the study, using only well matched pairs in both groups. Corneal graft survival of these two groups, both well matched for HLA-A and -B demonstrate again a lower, but not significant (overall p=0.07) graft survival for the eyes enucleated because of M.C.M. (fig. 3), 79.5%, 71.5% and 63.2% for the donor eyes enucleated because of M.C.M. at one, two and three years versus 94.5%, 87.0% and 81.5% for the others at the same time interval. These differences are most apparent during the first 9 months of follow-up. Just as in fig. 2 there was a large excess of failures in the M.C.M. donor group (O/E=1.381) as compared to the systemic malignancies group (O/E=0.564). Again, we tabulated the negative and positive influences on corneal graft survival in these two groups. Table 2 shows that there were no significant differences with regard to factors influencing corneal graft survival of corneas from donors deceased of a systemic malignancy versus the patient group with corneas from enucleated eyes because of M.C.M.

The influence of the initial disease in the recipient cornea on the fate of the corneal graft survival has been reported in chapter 5. Fig. 4 in that chapter demonstrates the poor survival of grafts in patients with the diagnosis

Table 2. Factors influencing corneal graft survival in donor-recipient pairs, well matched for HLA-A and -B

	Grafts from donors deceased of systemic malignancies (N=42)		Grafts from eyes enucleated because of M.C.M. (N=40)	
NEGATIVE				
- previous graft failures	30	(71.4%)	25	(62.5%)
- vascularised recipients	38	(90.4%)	35	(87.5%)
- large corneal graft diameter	18	(42.8%)	16	(40.4%)
POSITIVE				
- female donor - female recipient combination	10	(23.8%)	6	(15.0%)
- HLA-A and -B matching	42	(100%)	40	(100%)

secondary Fuchs dystrophy (S.F.U.C.). In table 3, the initial diseases are listed for the two donor cornea malignancy classes (systemic malignancies and choroidal melanomas). There is an excess of patients with secondary Fuchs' dystrophy (or secondary endothelial decompensation = S.E.D.) in the group of patients who received corneas from donors deceased from systemic malignancies (X^2=7.17, p=0.01). Paradoxically, the survival of the 42 grafts from donors with systemic malignancies,which include 13 patients with secondary endothelial decompensation (S.E.D.) is better than the

Table 3. Initial disease in the recipient corneas in HLA-A and -B well matched grafts from donors deceased of systemic malignancies and grafts from donor eyes enucleated because of a malignant choroidal melanoma (M.C.M.)

Initial disease of the recipient cornea	Grafts from donors deceased of systemic malignancies (N=42)	Grafts from eyes enucleated because of M.C.M. (N =40)
Keratoconus	3	4
Primary Fuchs (P.E.D.)	1	5
Named dystrophy	1	3
Miscellaneous	1	1
Trauma	3	2
Herpes	19	20
Burns	1	2
Secondary Fuchs (S.E.D.)	13*	3*

The factors have been ranked according to increasing levels of adverse effect on graft survival
* Levels of secondary Fuchs' patients were significantly different ($X^2 = 7.17$, uncorrected $p < 0.01$)

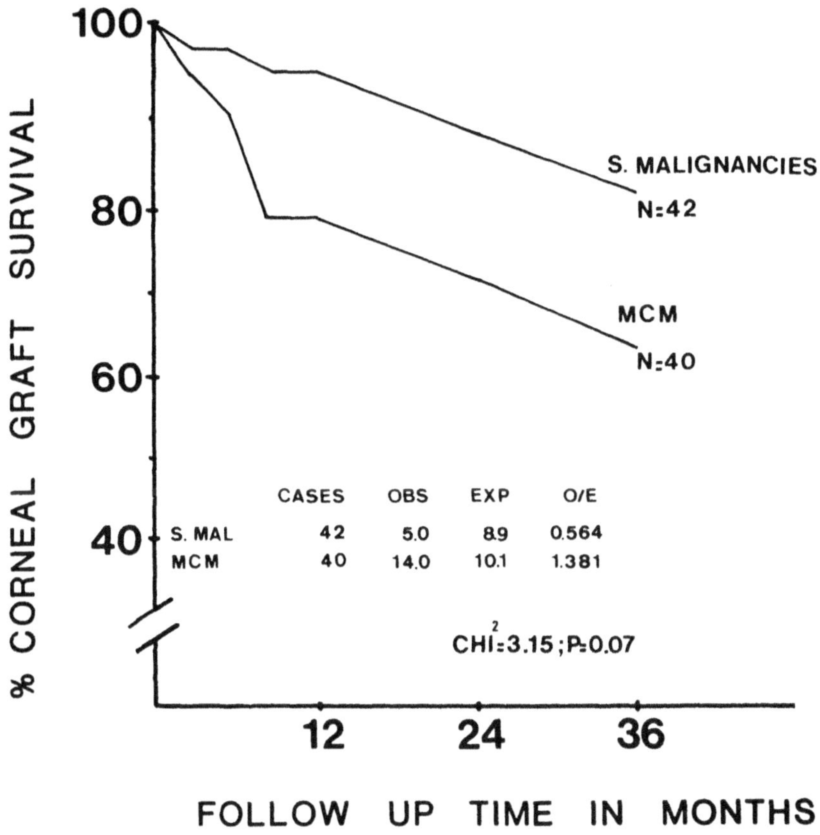

Figure 3. Analysis of the survival of HLA-A and -B matched corneal grafts from donors deceased of systemic malignancies (S.MAL) and from eyes enucleated because of a malignant choroidal melanoma (MCM).

survival of the 40 grafts from donor eyes enucleated because of M.C.M. (fig. 3), which is contrary to expectation.

The interval between 'death' and enucleation was of course zero in the eyes enucleated because of M.C.M., the interval between 'death' and transplantation was 1 to 70 hours with an average of 18.3 hours. In the group of donors with systemic malignancies the interval between death and enucleation was 3 to 16 hours with an average of 11.3 hours and the interval between death and transplantation was 6 to 81 hours with an average of 32.3 hours.

In table 4, the causes of graft failure for the two groups of HLA-A and -B well matched grafts are listed. The number of irreversible rejections is significantly higher (X^2=5.0, p=0.03) in the group of donor corneas from eyes enucleated because of M.C.M.

Table 4. Causes of graft failure in HLA-A and -B well matched grafts from donors deceased of systemic malignancies and in grafts from donor eyes enucleated because of a malignant choroidal melanoma (M.C.M.)

Cause of graft failure	Grafts from donors deceased of systemic malignancies (N=42)	Grafts from eyes enucleated because of M.C.M. (N=40)
- Irreversible rejection	3*	11*
- Glaucoma	3	2
- Infection/herpes recurrence	2	3
- Deficient tear production	1	3
- Insufficient donor material	2	0
- Trauma	2	1
Deceased	0	2
(still functioning)	29	18

* Numbers of irreversible rejections were significantly different ($X^2 = 5.002$, uncorrected $p = 0.03$)

Discussion

Neither the survival of corneal grafts obtained from eyes enucleated because of malignant choroidal melanoma nor a comparison of their survival with that of grafts from donors deceased of systemic malignancies have been reported previously.

The corneas of eyes enucleated because of a M.C.M. were the only source of donor material between 1939 and 1946 in Holland (chapter 3). There are no case reports in the literature of malignant melanoma being transferred in this manner (Paufique 1950, Kok-van Alphen 1950, King 1972, De Voe 1975). After 1946, information about the use of cadaveric donor material became available and shortage of donor eyes with M.C.M. stimulated the use of cadaveric donor corneas.

The use of corneas from donors deceased because of systemic malignancies, if a careful selection procedure is undertaken, is not contraindicated (Wagoner et al. 1981).

When we started HLA matching for corneal grafts in 1976 tissue typing of living donors, with intraocular tumors, was more reliable than the typing of blood from cadaveric donors. At that time, there were frequently prolonged delays between the collection of donor blood samples and their transport to the typing laboratories. Therefore, corneas from eyes enucleated because of M.C.M. were used for transplantation purposes once again.

When we first analysed the grafts performed in the period between January 1976 and April 1980, we observed a tendency of a lower graft survival in grafts obtained from eyes enucleated because of a M.C.M.

Therefore, we stopped the use of those donor corneas after June 1980. It took us from April 1976 until the end of December 1982 to collect sufficient HLA-A and -B matched corneal grafts from donors deceased of a systemic malignancy. Since we did not change our surgical technique nor the postoperative treatment in the period under review, we were able to compare the transplantation results in the two patient groups. The lower level of graft survival of the 44 corneal grafts obtained from eyes enucleated because of M.C.M. as compared to the 158 grafts from donors deceased from a systemic malignancy could not be explained by an excess of negative influences on corneal graft survival in the M.C.M. group. The high degree of HLA-A and -B matched grafts (90.9%) in this latter group was combined with an increased amount of vascularised recipient corneas (84.0%) because HLA-A and -B matching was restricted to vascularised corneasand/or previous rejections. In order to avoid these differences a selection of HLA-A and -B matched cases for both groups was made. Again, the lower graft survival of donor corneas obtained from eyes enucleated because of M.C.M. was observed. Analysis of the negative and positive influences on corneal graft survival in these censored groups revealed no significant differences, and those factors, therefore, are not sufficient to explain the difference in corneal graft survival. The influence of the patients' initial diseases on corneal graft survival is known; keratoconus patients always have a better graft survival as compared to those with herpes keratitis or alkaline burns. The graft survival for the various initial disease classes in our patients is presented in chapter 5. The lower graft survival for the donor corneas obtained from eyes enucleated because of M.C.M. cannot be explained by the influence of the initial disease. On the contrary, a significant excess of secondary Fuchs patients was observed in the group of corneas from donors with systemic malignancy. Even though this diagnosis class has the poorest graft survival of all diagnoses, the grafts from these donors deceased of systemic malignancies survived better than those from M.C.M. donors.

Although we could not detect a significant influence of the time interval between donor death and enucleation or donor death and transplantation on corneal graft survival (chapter 5). Polack (1977) recommends short time intervals. Since the 'death to enucleation interval' is zero in eyes enucleated because of M.C.M. and the 'death' to transplantation interval was an average of 18.3 hours, while the intervals were 11.3 hours and 32.3 hours respectively for the corneas obtained from patients deceased of a systemic malignancy, a lower level of graft survival in grafts obtained from eyes enucleated because of M.C.M. was not expected.

Conclusions

The causes of graft failure in the two study groups were not significantly different for all other causes except for irreversible rejection. The number of irreversible rejections in the group of eyes enucleated because of M.C.M. was significantly elevated. No explanation for this observation is available. There are no reports in the literature on this subject. One possibility is that the intraocular malignant choroidal melanoma alters some immunological properties of the donor eye, and this is a subject for further study.

Acknowledgements

We wish to thank Mrs. D. de Wolff-Rouendaal of the Department of Ophthalmology for the histological examination of the donor eyes containing a malignant choroidal melanoma and the staff of the typing and screening laboratories of the Department of Immunohaematology of the Leyden University Hospital for the excellent technical help.

References

Harms, H. and Mackensen, H. (1966) Augenoperationen unter dem Mikroskop. Thieme Verlag, Stuttgart, p 291.

King, J.H. (1972) Eyebank and the availability of corneas in the causes of preventness of blindness. Proc. series, Jerusalem seminar. ed. J.C. Michaelson, E.R. Berman. Academic Press, New York, 273.

Kok-van Alphen, C.C. (1954) Bijdrage tot de keratoplastiek. Diss. Eduard IJdo, Leiden, p 55.

Paufique, M. (1948) Les greffes de la cornée. Masson, Paris, 70.

Peto, R., Pike, M.C., Armitage, P., Breslow, N.E., Cox, D.R., Howard, S.V., Mantel, N., McPherson, K., Peto, J. and Smith, P.G. (1976) Design and analysis of randomized clinical trials recognizing prolonged observation of each patient. J.Br.J. Cancer 34: 585.

Polack, F.M. (1977) Corneal Transplantation. New York, Grune and Stratton, 98-99.

Rood van, J.J. (1979) Microlymphocytotoxicity method. In: NIAID manual of tissue typing techniques (Ed: S. Ray) National Institutes of Health (NIH) (80-545) Maryland, U.S.A.: 104.

De Voe, A.G. (1975) Complications of keratoplasty. The Gifford Lecture. Am.J.Ophthamol. 79: 907-912.

Völker-Dieben, H.J.M., Kok-van Alphen, C.C., Lansbergen, Q. and Persijn, G.G. (1982) Different influences on corneal graft survival in 539 transplants. Acta Ophthalm. 60: 190-202.

Wagoner, M.D., Dohlman, C.H., Albert, D.M., Lavin, P., Murphy, A., O'Neill-Dryja, M. (1981) Corneal donor selection. Ophthalmology vo. 88, 2, 139-144

SECTION II

Factors which may influence corneal graft survival

CHAPTER 5

Different influences on corneal graft survival in 539 transplants*

Summary

Different factors influencing the survival of 539 corneal grafts were studied. Their follow-up periods ranged from 3 months to 4½ years. The degree of vascularization of the host corneas, previous graft failures and the diameter of the grafts influenced the graft survival significantly. A significant influence of sex differences between donors and recipients was also observed. Grafts from female donors result in a better graft survival in female recipients as compared to male recipients. No significant influence on graft survival was found for pregnancies and blood transfusions. We could not find a significant influence of age of the donor, storage methods and time interval up to 78 hours between death and transplantation.

Introduction

Corneal transplants fail or become opaque for several different reasons. The most common cause of early graft failure in penetrating corneal transplants was defective endothelium on the donor cornea and/or defective wound closure resulting in a flat anterior chamber. Careful donor cornea selection and improved surgical technique, due to the introduction of the operating microscope and monofil nylon sutures, has reduced the early graft failure to an extremely rare event. Unfortunately however, the same cannot be said of intermediate or late corneal graft failure.

We decided to analyze different factors influencing corneal graft survival in a group of 539 full thickness keratoplasties. Neither the surgical technique nor the postoperative treatment has been changed during the period of the study. The aim of this study was to establish the positive and negative factors influencing corneal graft survival.

Material and methods

From January 1976 until April 1980, 539 full thickness keratoplasties were performed. The follow-up period ranged from 3 months to 4½ years.

All survival times were calculated using the actuarial life table method.

* *For colour plates, see pp. 72ff.*

The significance of the differences between the various classes were tested with X^2 statistics derived from log rank test (Peto et al. 1976). The numbers to the right of the follow-up curves (fig. 1 to 7) indicate the numbers of patients at risk at the start of the study.

The number of grafts performed in the successive years 1976 to May 1980 are summarized in table 1. Of the total of 539 grafts, 352 were first transplants. The number of single and repeated grafts are summarized in table 2.

Table 1. The number of grafts per year

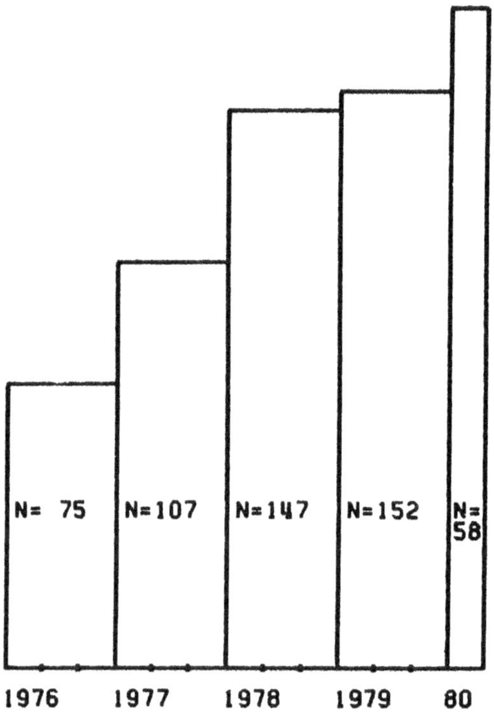

Table 2. The number of single and repeated grafts

First graft	N=352
Second graft	N=112
Third graft	N= 40
Fourth graft	N= 22
Fifth graft	N= 7
Sixth graft and more	N= 6
	N=539

Table 3. The initial indication for grafting

Diagnosis	Number of cases
Herpetic keratitis	194
Fuchs endothelial dystrophy	118
Keratoconus	64
Other dystrophies	26
Injuries	19
Burns	19
Others	99
Total	539

The initial indications for grafting are listed in table 3. The most common diameter of the graft is 7.5 mm (N=203). The diameter 7.0 (N=139) and the diameter 8.0 (N=133) ranking second and third respectively. Table 4 lists the graft diameters in the transplanted corneas.

All transplantations were performed by two surgeons (Völker-Dieben and Kok-van Alphen). Our surgical techniques were identical. The technique was according to the method described by Harms and Mackensen (1966). A running suture of 10x0 monofil nylon was used after 4 pre-placed sutures which were removed during operation.

In all cases, the postoperative treatment consisted of dexamethason 1% eyedrops, 3 times daily, combined with antibiotic eyedrops, for at least one year. No systemic steroid therapy nor immune suppressive therapy was given to the patients.

Corneal donor material was selected on the quality of the morphological picture of the endothelial cells by means of slit-lamp examination and specular microscopy. Corneal donor material was either stored in McCarey Kaufman tissue culture medium (N=295) or taken directly from the globe as described in detail elsewhere (Rycroft 1955) (N=244) and used within 24 h after death.

Table 4. Graft diameter in mm

Graft diameter in mm	Number of grafts
<7.0	18
7.0	139
7.5	203
8.0	133
8.5	31
>9.0	15
Total	539

In case of storage, the donor cornea was punched on a teflon block, endothelial side up. Table 5 shows the number of hours between the death of the donor and transplantation. The maximum time interval has been 78 hours.

Table 5. Time between death and transplantation in hours

0– 9 h	N= 63
10–19 h	N= 77
20–29 h	N= 91
30–39 h	N= 42
40–49 h	N= 83
50–59 h	N= 23
>59 h	N= 17
Unknown	N=143
Total	N=539

The age of the donors ranged from 8 to 96 years (see table 6).

Table 6. Age of the donor

<45	N=108
46–60	N=106
61–75	N=142
76–90	N= 87
>90	N= 2
Unknown	N= 94
Total	N=539

The causes of death of the donors were reported in 371 cases. A sudden death was caused by heart failure (N=106), cerebro vascular accident (N=45) and a road traffic accident (N=55). Carcinoma (not of the eye) was the cause of death in 100 cases. These data are summarized in table 7.

The sex of the donor was known in 432 cases, 261 male and 171 female donors. The recipients consisted of 295 male and 244 female patients. 140 Male patients received a male donor cornea and 80 female patients received a

Table 7. Causes of death of the donor

Heart failure	N=106
Carcinoma	N=100
C.V.A.	N= 45
Accident	N= 55
Miscellaneous	N= 65
Total	N=371

female donor cornea. The distribution of the sex of donors and recipients is shown in table 8.

Table 8. Sex distribution of donors and recipients

		RECIPIENT	
		Male	Female
DONOR	Male	140	119
	Female	91	80

ABO blood groups were known for 178 donors and 332 recipients. The distribution of the ABO blood groups of donors and recipients is shown in table 9. Ninety three donors and 164 recipients were blood group A, 60 donors and 142 recipients were blood group O. AB blood group was found in 8 donors and 7 recipients, B was found in 17 donors and 19 recipients.

Table 9. ABO Blood groups of donor and recipient

	A	B	AB	O	?	Total
Donor	93	17	8	60	361	539
Recipient	164	19	7	142	207	539

Table 10 shows the distribution of the A and O blood groups in 134 donor and recipient combinations. Due to the small numbers of AB and B donors and recipients, it was decided not to investigate these 2 groups separately.

Fifty blood group A recipients received corneas from A donors and 28 O recipients received corneas from O donors. In 32 cases, there was ABO incompatibility between the recipients and cornea donors. The remaining 24 cases were ABO compatible, but not identical.

Table 10. Distribution of A and O blood groups in 134 donor-recipient combinations

		RECIPIENT	
		A	O
DONOR	A	50	32
	O	24	28

Information was collected concerning the number of blood transfusions the patient had received before the date of the corneal graft as well as concerning the number of pregnancies and abortions of the female recipients. The information was mostly collected via personal interviews by one of us (Völker-Dieben). A few patients provided the information by means of a written questionnaire.

Table 11 summarizes the data concerning the number of blood transfusions. 353 Patients received 0 transfusions and only 3 patients had had more than 5 transfusions. The number of transfusions was unknown in 112 patients.

Table 11. Number of recipient blood transfusions

Transfusions	0	1	2–4	⩾5	?	Total
Recipients	353	29	42	3	112	539

The information about pregnancies and abortions of 244 female patients is summarized in table 12. 65 Females had never been pregnant, 20 females were once pregnant, 88 females had 2 to 4 pregnancies and 29 females had 5 or more pregnancies. No information could be obtained from 42 female patients.

Table 12. Number of pregnancies and abortions of 244 female recipients

Pregnancies	0	1	2–4	⩾5	?	Total
Recipients	65	20	88	29	42	244

Vascularisation of the recipient cornea at the time of transplantation and previous graft rejections are important predictors of graft clarity. The vascularisation levels of the recipient corneas were divided into four grades, 1: none ○, 2: slight ⦶, 3: moderate –⊕–, 4: severe ✳ (See colour plate 1). In order to simplify the comparison with the work of Gibbs et al. (1974), we used the same criteria and symbols for assigning the degree of vascularisation - non, slight, moderate and severe - of the host cornea.

Table 13 shows the vascularisation grades of the recipient corneas. No vessels were found in 20 recipient corneas, 169 corneas were considered to be slightly vascularized. 119 Corneas were moderately vascularized and 209 severely. The degree of vascularization grade was not described for 22 recipient corneas.

Table 13. The level of vascularisation of the recipient corneas

Grade						
Vascularisation	None	Slight	Moderate	Severe	?	Total
Recipients	20	169	119	209	22	539

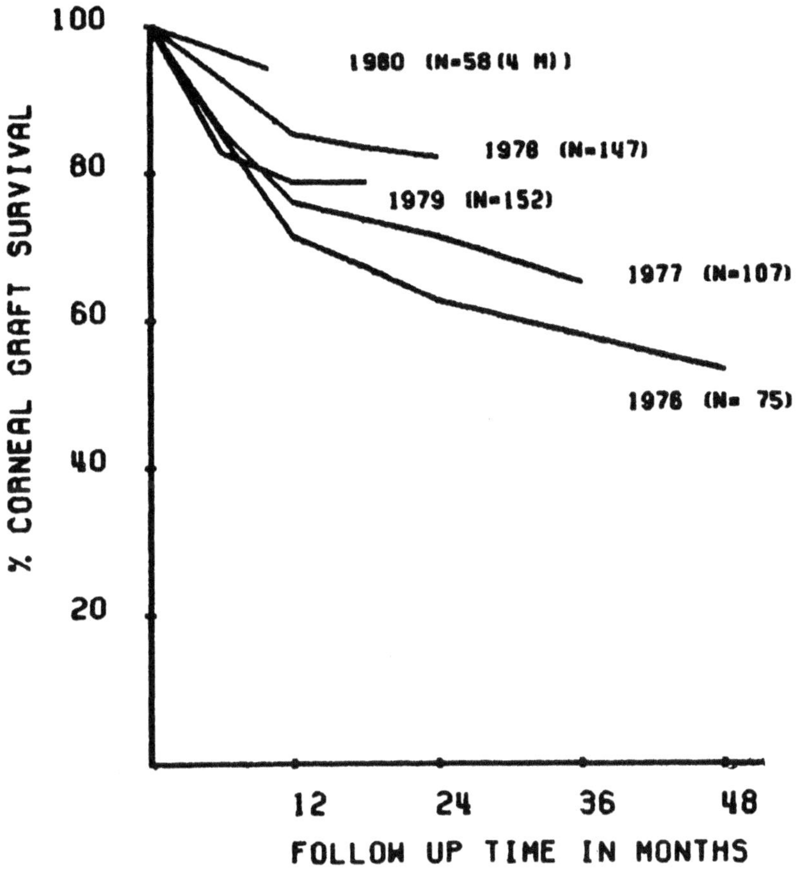

Figure 1. Corneal graft survival per year.

Results

Fig. 1 shows that corneal graft survival was not significantly influenced by the cause of death of the donors (overall p=0.27). However, donors recorded with the diagnosis carcinoma consisted of individuals whose eyes were enucleated because of M.C.M. as well as those who died from systemic malignancies. The survival of grafts from donors in these two classes covered by the diagnosis 'carcinoma' (fig. 2) was not significantly different (overall p=0.08). However, inspection of the two curves reveals that they essentially overlap up to 9 months post transplantation. Thereafter, they diverge, with the donor corneas from eyes enucleated because of M.C.M. showing a lower graft survival than those from individuals who died because of systemic malignancies.

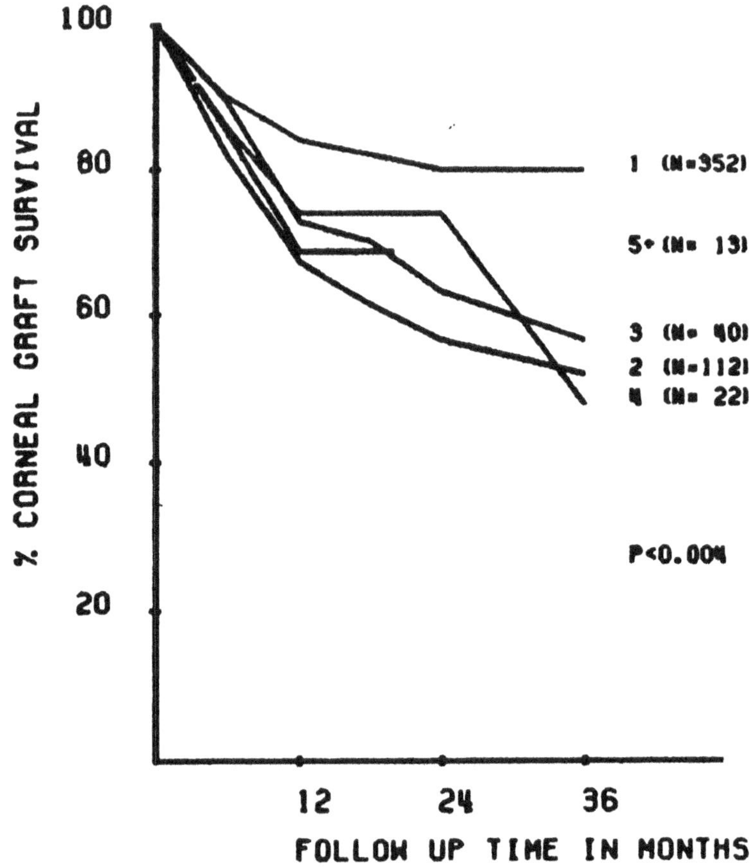

Figure 2. Influence of previous graft failures.

The graft survival rates in moderately and severely vascularized corneas are not significantly different from each other.

The effect of the initial disease before grafting on graft survival is shown in fig. 4. Recipients with an initial diagnosis of keratoconus have a very much better survival than recipients in the other diagnostic groups.

The diameter of the graft was found to have a significant effect on the graft survival. If the graft diameter increases, the graft survival rate decrease ($p<0.005$). Fig. 5 shows a graft survival rate of 82% in the group of patients who received a corneal graft with a diameter between 7.0 and 8.4 mm. The graft survival rate was 57% and 56% respectively after one year in the group of patients who received a corneal graft with a diameter between 8.5 to 8.9 and 9.0 mm and more, respectively.

The influence of sex differences between the donors and recipients are

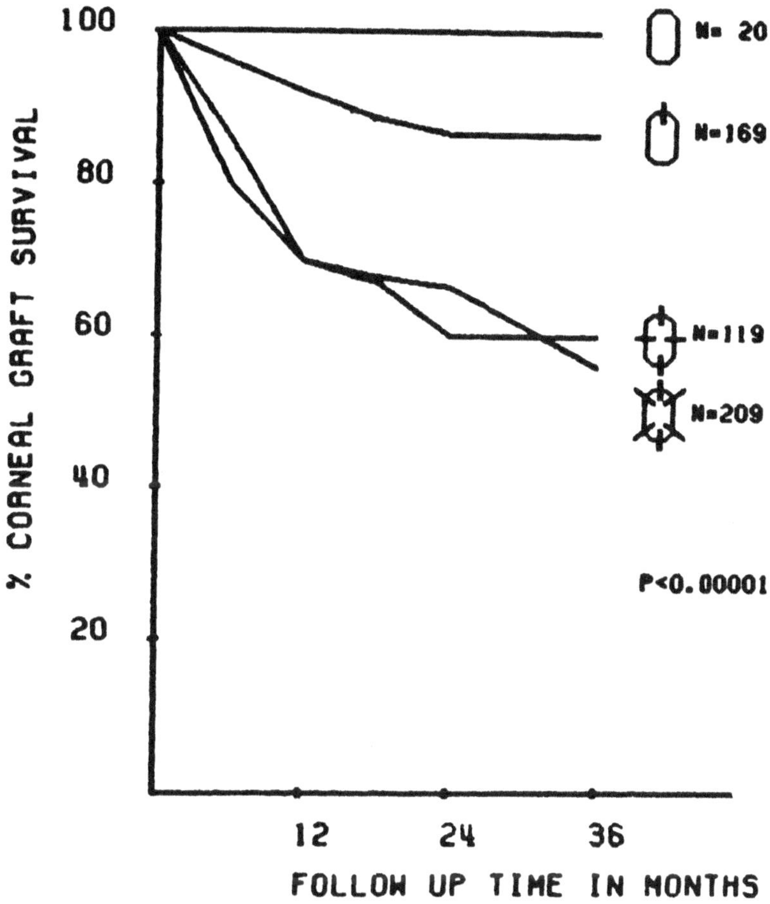

Figure 3. Influence of vascularisation.

shown in fig. 6. A female donor cornea results in a better graft survival in female recipients, 85% survival at one year compared to male recipients who have 76% at one year. Hereafter,no more differences are observed between the two groups. However, grafts from male donors do not significantly influence graft survival in male recipients, 79% at one year, compared to female recipients, 80% at one year (data not shown).

O recipients who received an A donor cornea had a better graft survival after one year (89%) as compared to A recipients who received an A donor cornea (74%), however, the differences were not significant (fig. 7). A recipients who received an O donor also showed no significant difference in graft survival, 85% at one year, as compared to O recipients who received an O cornea donor 90% (data not shown). Therefore, O recipients do as well

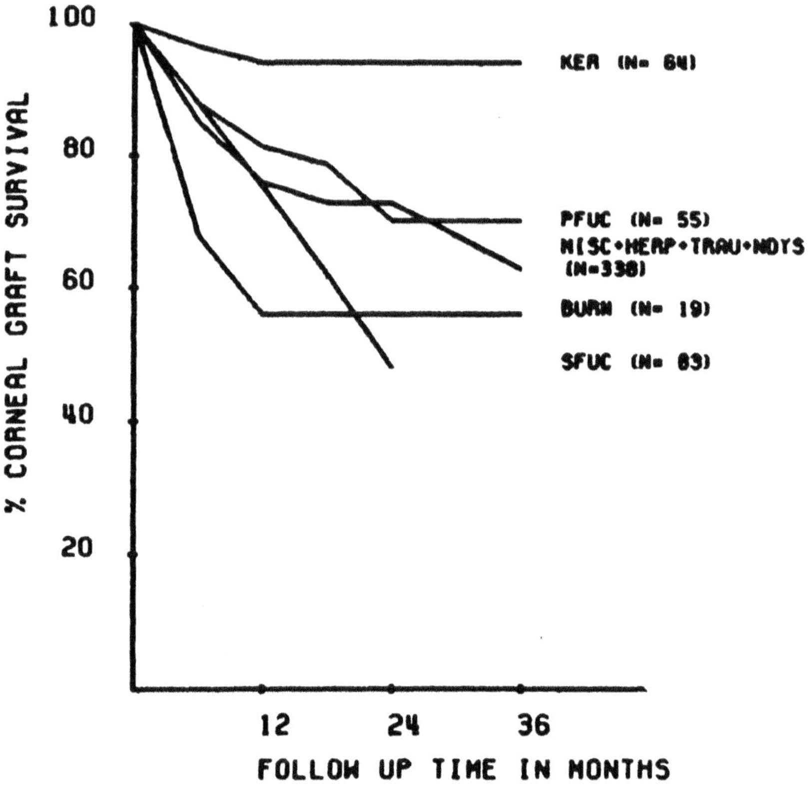

Figure 4. Influence of the initial disease.

with corneas from blood group A and blood group O donors.

No significant influence of pregnancies or blood transfusions were found, neither in the total material nor in the highly vascularized corneas only, with and without exclusion of the non immunological failures. These findings are not in concordance with the observations in kidney transplantation (Persijn et al. 1979).

No significant differences in graft survival were found among the different methods for storage of the donor material, nor with the time interval between death of the donor and transplantation. Neither the age of the donor nor the cause of death seemed to influence graft survival.

Discussion

The negative influence of previous failures on graft survival rates as suggested by the work of Gibbs et al. (1974) and Khodadoust (1979), was

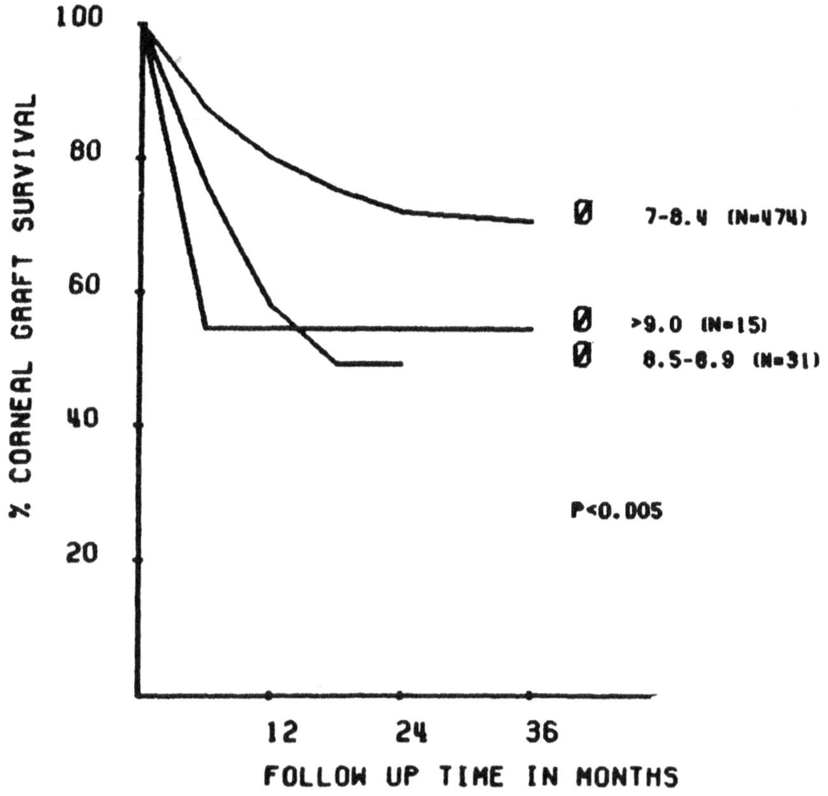

Figure 5. Influence of the graft diameter.

demonstrated to be statistically significant in the whole material of 539 grafts as well as in the group of vascularized corneas only. Another known negative influence on the corneal graft survival rate, the degree of vascularization (Khodadoust 1973; Batchelor et al. 1976), was also found to be statistically significant. (p=0.00001). Since graft failures attract blood vessel ingrowth, those 2 negative influences are not mutually exclusive.

Although Nelkens (1956) was the first to describeABO antigens were in the cornea, Herold (1972) found that the ABO antigens located only in the epithelial layer of the cornea. The influence of ABO blood groups on graft survival was described by Mailäth et al. (1972). A better graft survival was found when donor and recipient were ABO compatible, as compared to when they were incompatible. Unfortunately, no subdivisions into different risk groups were made. Meyer (1971) did not find any influence of ABO compatibilities on corneal graft survival.

The influence of host and donor sex has, to our knowledge, not yet been described in human corneal grafts. Van Vreeswijk and Balner (1980)

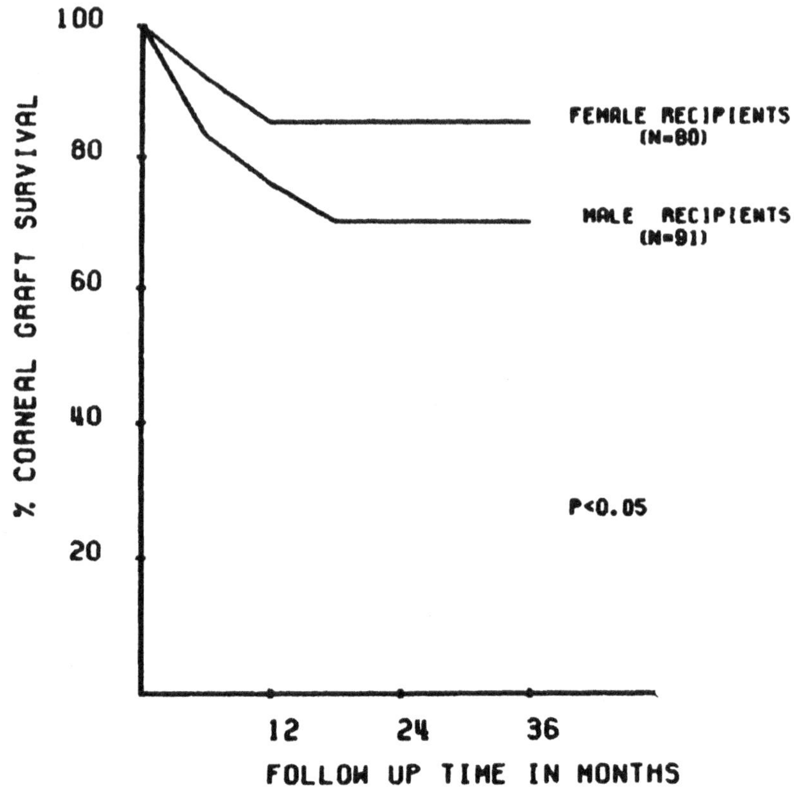

Figure 6. Influence of female donor.

described a possible influence of host and donor sex in skin allografts in rhesus monkeys. They observed that grafts from female donors were rejected more rapidly by female recipients. Our observation in man of a better corneal graft survival rate in female donor - female recipient combinations is not in concordance with their findings in skin grafts in monkeys.

There was an inverse correlation between corneal graft diameter and graft survival ($p<0.005$). Grönemeyer (1976) showed, in inbred rats, that the number of corneal graft rejections is significantly increased if the graft reached the limbal region. Our results, in man, agree with his experimental results. If the graft reaches the limbal vessels, the possibility of encountering cytotoxic cells increases. In addition, if previous graft failures had occurred the next graft will be larger than the previous one in order to excise all clouded corneal material. The adverse effect of large corneal graft diameter is not seen in keratoconus patients who almost always have avascular corneas.

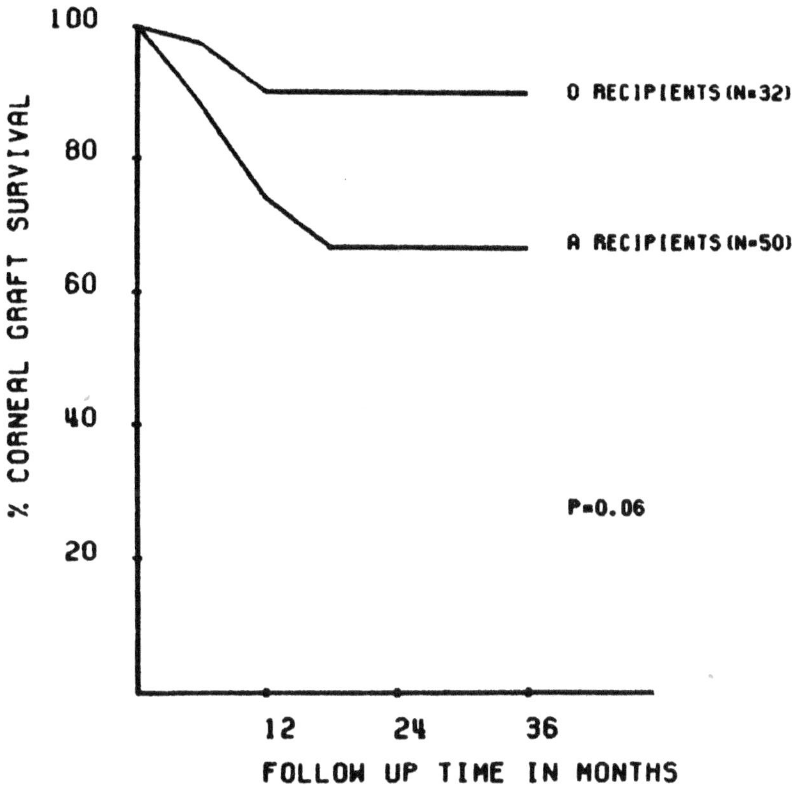

Figure 7. Influence of bloodgroup A donor.

Conclusion

In 539 corneal grafts, we could distinguish several factors which influence corneal graft survival. Negative influences:
1. previous graft failures;
2. high degree of corneal vascularization;
3. large corneal graft diameter.

Possible positive influence:
1. A donor - O recipient combinations;
2. female donor -female recipient combinations.

No influences:
1. pregnancies;
2. blood transfusions;
3. donor age;
4. cause of death of the donor;
5. time interval between death of donor and transplantation (0-72 h);
6. storage methods.

ACKNOWLEDGEMENTS

This study could not have been conducted without the generous support and cooperation of the theatre staff of the Leyden University Eye Clinic, without which the 539 corneal grafts could not have been performed.

We wish to thank the staff of the Department of Immunohaematology of the Leyden University Hospital for their excellent technical help.

References

Batchelor J.R., Casey T.A., Gibbs D.C., Loyd D.F., Werb A., Prasad S.S. and James A. (1976) HLA matching and corneal grafting. Lancet 1: 551-554.

Gibbs D.C., Batchelor J.R., Werb A., Schlesinger W. and Casey T.A. (1974) The influence of tissue typing compatibility on the rate of full-thickness corneal grafts. Trans. Ophthal. Soc. U.K. 94: 101-109.

Grönemeyer U., Pülhorn G. and Müller-Ruchholtz W. (1976) Histoincompatibility and allogeneic corneal grafting between inbred strains of rats. Mod. Probl. Ophthalmol. 16: 161.

Harms H. and Mackensen H. (1966) Augenoperationen unter dem Mikroskop, pp. 291. Thieme Verlag, Stuttgart.

Herold W. (1972) Zum Nachweis der Blutgruppenantigene A und B in der menschlichen Hornhaut mittels der Immunfluoreszenstechnik. Klin. Monatsbl. Augenheilkd. 161: 658.

Khodadoust A.A. (1973) The allograft rejection reaction: The leading cause of late failure of clinical corneal grafts. In: Corneal Graft Failure. Ciba Found. Symp. 15: 151. Associated Scientific Publishers, Amsterdam/London/New York.

Khodadoust A.A. and Abizedeh A. (1979) The fate of corneal grafts after previous rejection reactions. Doc. Ophthalmol. Proc. Ser. 20: 115-122.

Kok-van Alphen C.C. and Völker-Dieben H.J.M. (1980) Impairment of tear production in corneal herpetic diseases. In Herpetische Augenerkrankungen 215-218, J.F. Bergman Verlag, München

Mailäth L., Stenszky V., Alberth B. and Aszödi L. (1972) Die Rolle der Blutgruppen-kompatibilität bei Keratoplastik. Klin. Monatsbl. Augenheilkd. 160: 550-553.

Meyer H.J. (1971) Spielen Blutfaktoren eine Rolle bei der Hornhauttransplantation? Dtsch. Med. Wochenschr. 96: 1259-1260.

Nelkens E., Michaelson J.C., Nelkens D. and Gurevitch J. (1956) ABO antigens in the human cornea. Nature 177: 840.

Persijn G.G., Cohen B., Lansbergen Q. and Van Rood J.J. (1979) Retrospective and prospective studies on the effect of blood transfusions in renal transplantation in The Netherlands. Transplantation 28: 396-401.

Peto R., Pike M.C., Armitage P., Breslow N.E., Cox D.R., Howard S.V., Mantel N., McPherson K., Peto J. and Smith P. (1976) Design and analysis of randomized clinical trials requiring prolonged observation of each patient. I. Br. J. Cancer 34: 585.

Rycroft B.W. (1955) Corneal grafts, pp. 172-173. Butterworth, London.

Van Vreeswijk W. and Balner H. (1980) Major histocompatibility complex matching and other factors influencing skin allograft survival in related and unrelated Rhesus monkeys. Transplantation 30: 196-202.

CHAPTER 6

The effect of prospective HLA-A and -B matching on corneal graft survival*

Summary

The effect of prospective HLA-A and -B matching on corneal graft survival was studied in 159 Dutch recipients. The follow-up period ranged from 3 months to 4½ years. In the same period, 380 grafts were performed without HLA matching. The influence of HLA-A and -B matching on graft survival in all vascularized cases (N=137) was significant (p=0.046). If the non-immunological failures were excluded the effect of HLA-A and -B matching became more pronounced (p=0.027). The influence of HLA-A and -B matching on the graft survival of only the first grafts in vascularized corneas is also significant (p=0.028). Finally a significant influence of HLA-A and -B matching was found in repeated grafts in vascularized corneas (p=0.037).

Introduction

Although in earlier times the cornea was thought to be poorly equipped to initiate immunological reactions, nowadays ophthalmologists know that the rejection of corneal grafts is a very important cause of graft failures.

Paufique (1948) was the first to describe the 'Maladie du Greffon', at that time an unexplained allergic phenomenon. That was, in fact, the first description of the clinical picture of graft rejection.

Maumenee (1951) studied the mechanism of tissue destruction when corneas were transplanted from one albino rabbit to another, followed by skin grafts from the same donor. The destruction was the result of a sensitization phenomena. He concluded that the reaction was not tissue specific, but individual specific.

Kok-van Alphen (1954) suggested that the recurrence of the herpes keratitis was the most important cause of graft failure. In 1979, the same author stated that corneal inflammation precipitated the immune reaction.

Vannas et al. (1970, 1976) were among the first to study the immunological aspects of corneal grafts. They observed a beneficial effect of antigen sharing between donor and recipient on corneal allograft survival.

Ehlers et al. (1971, 1973) and Gibbs et al. (1974) reported the influence of histocompatibility on the fate of corneal transplants. Their results, obtained from retrospectively HLA-typed corneal graft donors suggest that, for recipients with vascularized corneas and/or previous graft failures, selection of HLA-compatible donors is essential. The increasing knowledge of the importance of histocompatibility on corneal graft survival stimulated us to investigate the influence of prospective HLA-A and -B matching on corneal graft survival.

* *For colour plates, see pp. 72ff.*

Material and methods

From January 1976 until April 1980, 539 full thickness keratoplasties were performed. All patients and graft donors were of Dutch Caucasoid origin. The follow-up period ranged from 3 months to 4½ years. 159 Of these keratoplasties were performed in HLA-A and -B typed prospectively selected recipients. These patients received the best possible HLA matched corneal graft. More than 2 mismatches were not accepted. The remaining 380 grafts were performed without HLA matching. All HLA typings of the patients and donors were performed in the National Reference Center in Leyden (Department of Immunohaematology, University Hospital) with the Eurotransplant serum set which recognizes all official HLA and workshops A and B specificities. Tissue typing was performed with a standard microlymphocytotoxicity assay (Van Rood, 1979).

HLA-A and -B locus typing was performed on peripheral blood of patients. All HLA phenotypes and other relevant data such as ABO, sex, date of birth etc. were stored into the Eurotransplant computer. Tissue typing of the donor was performed on peripheral blood obtained within 2 hours after death, when the donor eyes were enucleated.

Tissue typing and matching was restricted to high risk cases, i.e. patients with severely vascularized corneas and/or previous corneal graft rejections. If no suitable recipient was available, the donor cornea was used at random. Tissue typing of the recipient was then performed retrospectively. The diagnosis of an immune allograft reaction is not always simple. It was summed up during the Ciba Symposium on corneal graft failure held in 1972 (see Ciba Foundation Symposium, 1973) as follows: an unequivocal clinical diagnosis of allograft reaction can be made when, at least 10 days after a first transplantation, a previously clear graft in a quiet eye rapidly develops oedema with signs of inflammation in the anterior segment including ciliary flush, with cells and usually a slight flare in the anterior chamber and when the area of oedema in the graft moves across the cornea in the wake of an endothelial line (Khodadoust rejection line). The same criteria were used for the diagnosis of an allograft reaction in repeated grafts (See colour plate 2, a and b).

All survival times were calculated using the actuarial life table method. The significance of the differences between the various classes were tested with X^2 statistics derived from the log rank test (Peto et al., 1976). The numbers to the right of the follow-up curves (fig. 1 to 6) indicate the numbers of patients at risk at the start of the study.

Results

We performed 159 grafts with HLA-A and -B matched donor material. The larger part (137 grafts) were performed in vascularized corneal beds. We

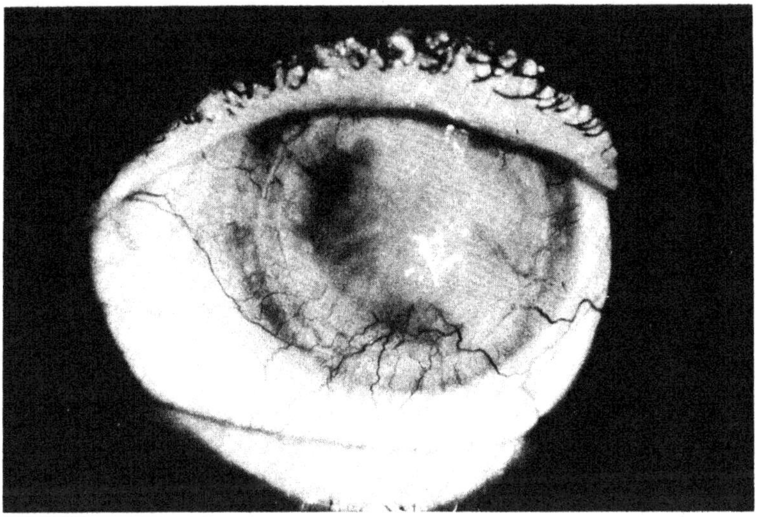

Figure 1a. Blood vessels are attracted by repeated grafts.

analyzed the complete material without any exclusions. No significant difference in corneal graft survival could be demonstrated in matched and not matched cases (fig. 1). However, the prognosis of the matched group is from the onset considerably less positive compared to the not matched group.

The graft survival was significantly influenced by the degree of vascularization and the number of previous graft failures. Since blood vessels are attracted by repeated grafts, these 2 features coincide (fig. 1a). For this reason, we were especially interested in the effect of HLA matching on graft survival in the vascularized corneas.

Of the 159 matched corneal grafts, 137 were used in vascularized corneas. The influence of HLA matching on the graft survival is set out in fig. 2. The overall results were only of borderline significance (p=0.046). The one year graft survival in the matched group is 76.1% versus 66.2% in the not matched group.

If we excluded the non-immunological failures (fig. 3) the effect of HLA-A and -B matching becomes more pronounced (p=0.027). The one year graft survival in the matched group is 88.3% versus 78.5% in the non matched group.

We could not demonstrate a clear cut correlation between the number of HLA mismatches and the graft survival in all cases (figure not shown). However, if we look to the influence of the number of mismatches in the highly vascularized corneas, we see a stepwise detoriation of the graft survival with increasing number of mismatches (fig. 4). Patients who received a 0 HLA mismatched corneal graft show a 91.1% graft survival after one year while patients who received a 2 HLA mismatched graft show a 85.4% graft

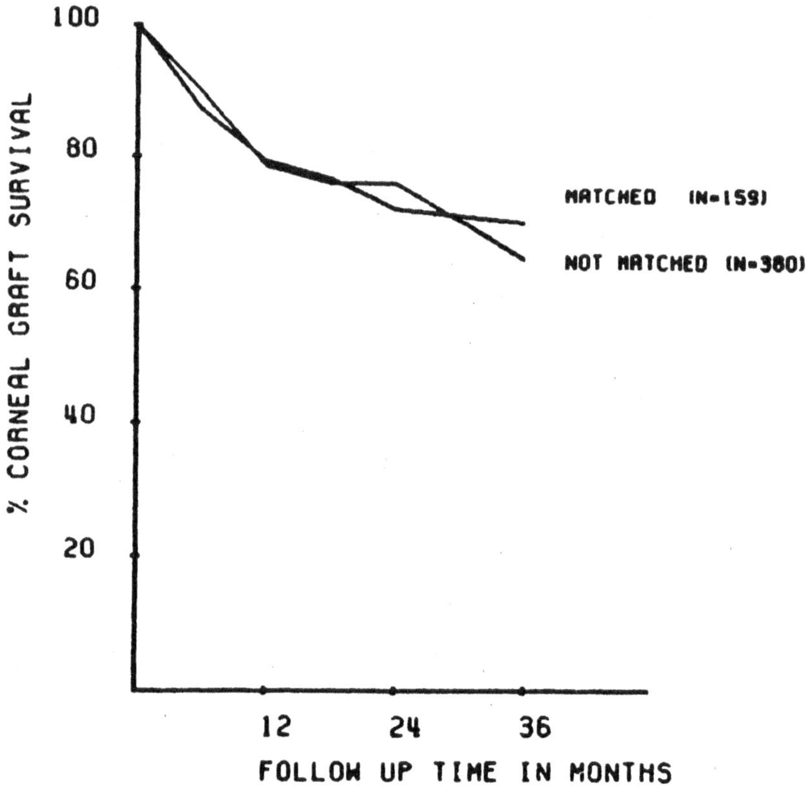

Figure 1. Influence of HLA-A and -B matching, no exclusions.

survival after one year. Patients who received a 1 HLA mismatched graft had an intermediate graft survival rate of 87.3% after one year. The number of patients at risk at 2 years for the HLA 0 mismatched corneal grafts was 4, for the 1 HLA mismatched grafts 11 and for the 2 HLA mismatched grafts 17. After 2 years, these numbers are still smaller, so no conclusions can be drawn and therefore the curves are indicated by dotted lines for that period in fig. 4.

Discussion

The selection of donor corneas on the basis of HLA-A and -B compatibility appears to increase the graft survival rate in vascularized corneas. Our findings confirm and extend our preliminary reports (Völker-Dieben et al., 1977, 1978) and the findings of Gibbs et al. (1979). In Gibbs' study, the influence of at least 2 HLA-A and -B antigens shared by donor and recipient had a beneficial effect on the graft survival rate in vascularized corneas

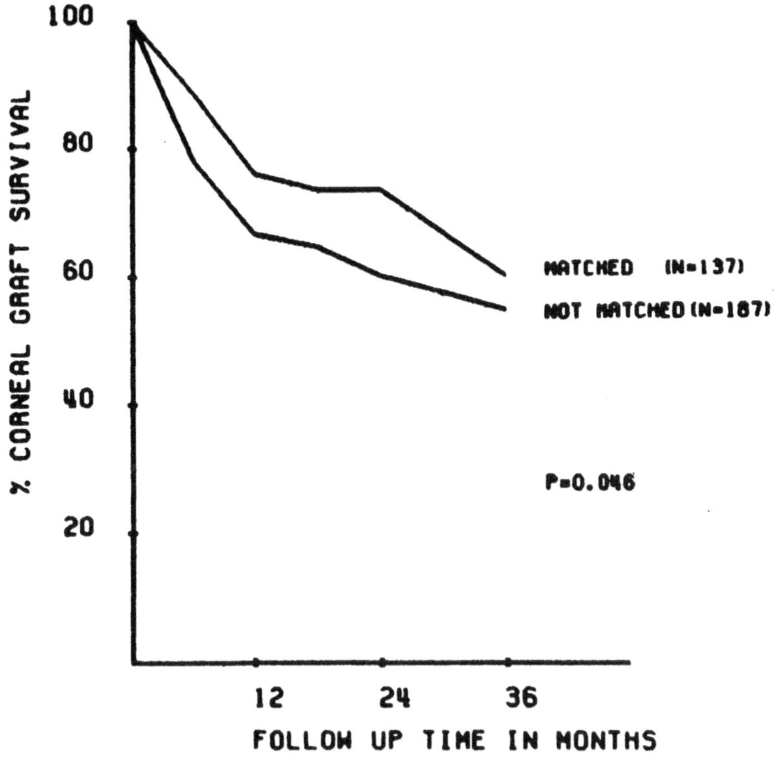

Figure 2. Influence of HLA-A and -B matching in vascularised corneas.

(N=44), although no statistical significance was reached. The same observations were reported by Ehlers and Kissmeyer-Nielsen (1979). In their study of 222 cases, the degree of vascularization of the recipient corneas was not reported. A significant decrease in the number of rejection episodes was found when the donor cornea shared at least two HLA-A, -B antigens with the recipient. However, if only the irreversible rejections were considered, the findings were no longer significant.

In our series of 137 prospectively well matched donor corneas and 187 non-matched donor corneas, both grafted in vascularized corneal beds by the same two surgeons during the same period, a statistically significant increase in graft survival was demonstrated (p=0.046) (fig. 2). If the non-immunological failures are excluded the significance is slightly better (p 0.027) (fig. 3).

An improved degree of graft survival correlated to the number of matched donor recipient antigens was found by Vannas et al. (1976) and Batchelor et al. (1976). However, Vannas did not divide her cases into different degrees of

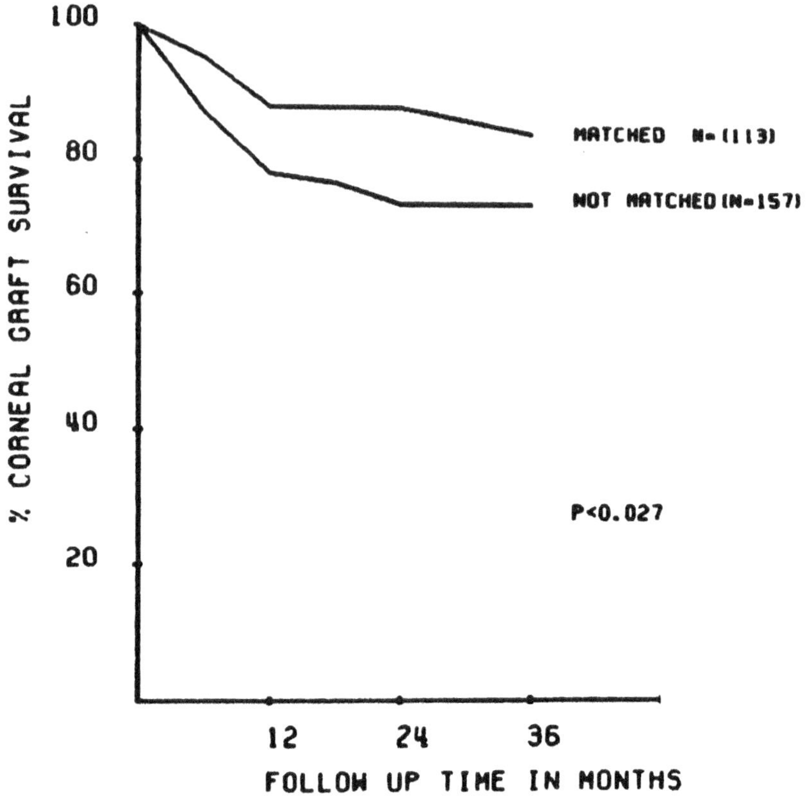

Figure 3. Influence of HLA-A and -B matching in vascularised corneas, non immunological failures excluded.

vascularization, and the series of Batchelor consisted of 73 keratoplasty recipients with dense corneal vascularization. Stark et al. (1979) could not confirm the beneficial effect of HLA matching in similar high risk cases. However, the majority of his cases received corneas from negatively cross matched donors. From a minority of our patients cross matching was known before grafting. No grafts were performed if a positive cross match was observed, however, the very small number of these patients does not influence the findings on the effect of HLA matching substantially.

The influence of the number of HLA mismatches in our material appears to be not significant if the vascularized corneas only are analyzed. The influence of the number of mismatches becomes clearer when non-immunological failures are excluded. Our series of 113 grafts in vascularized corneas (non-immunological failures excluded) reveals a negative influence of increasing number of mismatches on graft survival, although not statistically significant.

As confirmatory laboratory tests for corneal allograft rejection are not

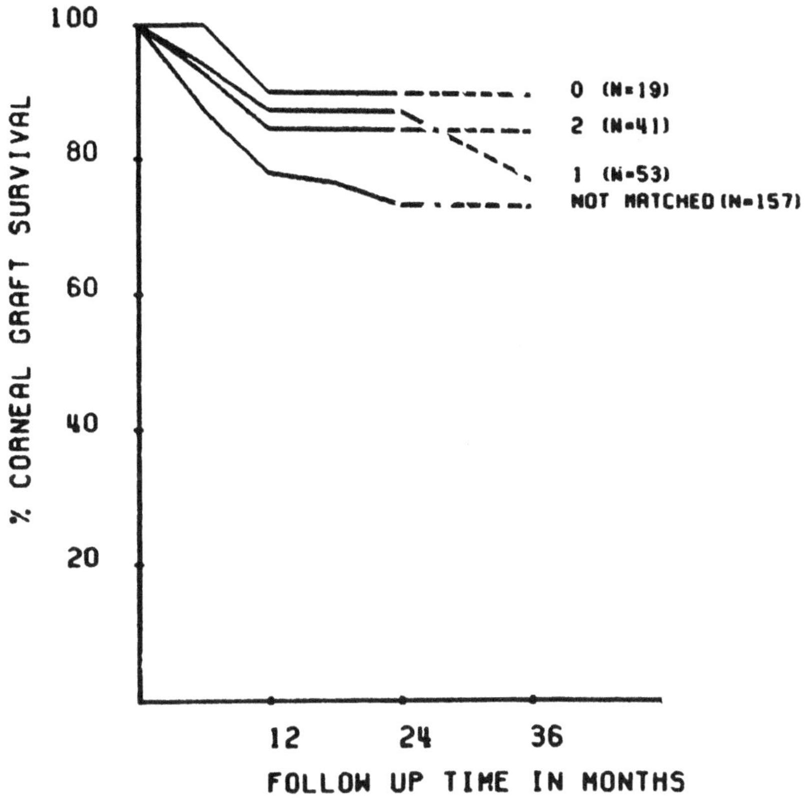

Figure 4. Influence of the number of HLA mismatches in vascularised corneas, non immunological failures excluded.

available, the diagnosis of graft rejection has to be made clinically. The tendency for improved graft survival with the use of HLA matched donor material for vascularized corneas found by Gibbs and Ehlers was confirmed and extended by our findings of a statistically significant improved graft survival rate with the use of HLA matched donor material.

Conclusion

We found a better corneal graft survival in the years following 1976. The percentage of matched grafts in vascularized corneas was only 10% in 1976 compared to 60% in 1977, 55% in 1978 and 50% in 1979 and 1980. The influence of HLA-A and -B matching per year was visible in a tendency to better graft survival in the matched group compared to the not matched group although not significant for each year separately.

A statistically significant negative influence on graft survival was demonstrated for repeated grafts; vascularized corneal beds and a large diameter of the graft (∅>8.4) (chapter 5).

A statistically significant positive influence on graft survival was found for female donor to female recipient combinations compared to female donor -male recipient combinations (chapter 5).

A possibly positive influence on graft survival was seen in blood group A donor - O recipient combinations compared to A donor - A recipient combinations (chapter 5). Analysis of these influences on the graft survival rate of the matched and not matched corneal grafts by means of cross tabulation revealed:

1. a strong association between matched grafts and repeat grafts ($p=0.00001$);
2. an association between repeat grafts and large grafts (∅>8.4) ($p=0.004$);
3. a negative association of female donor to female recipient combinations and matched grafts ($p=0.05$).

The high numbers of repeated and large grafts and the relatively low number of female donor - female recipient combinations exert 3 negative

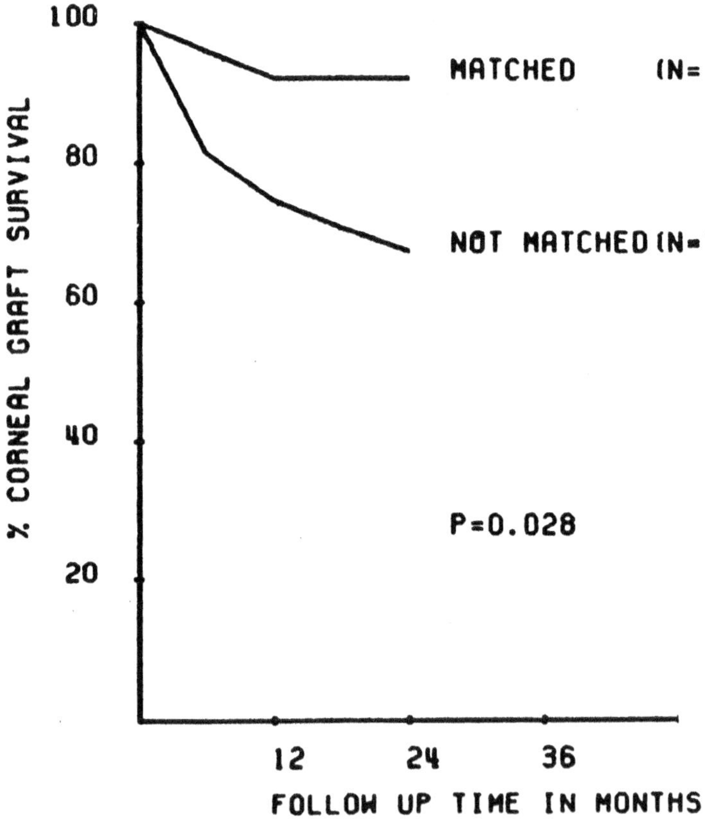

Figure 5. Influence of HLA-A and -B matching in vascularised corneas, first grafts.

influences on graft survival in the group of matched grafts. Blood group A donor to O recipient combinations were randomly distributed in the matched and not matched groups. The influence of HLA-A and -B matching on vascularized corneas in first grafts is shown in fig. 5. A significant influence of HLA-A and -B matching on corneal graft survival was found (p=0.028), 91.3% survival after one year in the matched group compared to 76.5% in the not matched group.

Fig. 6 shows the significant influence of HLA-A and -B matching in vascularized corneas and repeated grafts (p=0.037). The corneal graft survival in the matched group is 71% survival after one year compared to 52% in the not matched group.

In figs. 5 and 6, the data of the first year 1976 were excluded for reason of the low percentage of HLA matched grafts (only 10%) in this year as was mentioned earlier.

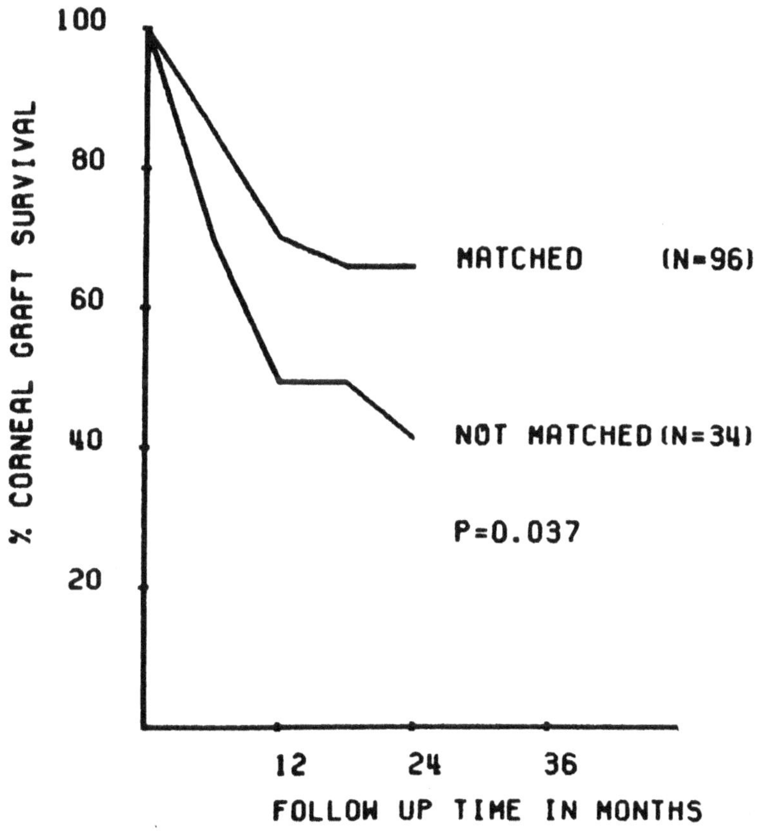

Figure 6. Influence of HLA-A and -B matching in vascularised corneas after one or more graft failures.

Our conclusion is that the selection of donors on the basis of HLA compatibility may result in a significantly better graft survival. We especially recommend HLA matched donor material for corneal grafts in patients with vascularized corneas and/or previous graft failures.

Acknowledgements

This study could not have been conducted without the generous support and cooperation of the theatre staff of the Leyden University Eye Clinic, without which the 539 corneal grafts could not have been performed.

We wish to thank Mr. P. de Lange for his help in the performance of the statistical analysis.

We also wish to thank the staff of the Departmentof Immunohaematology of the Leyden University Hospital and especially the tissue typing and screening laboratories for their excellent technical help.

References

Batchelor J.R., Casey T.A., Gibbs D.C., Lloyd D.F., Werb A., Prasad S.S. and James A. (1976) HLA-A matching and corneal grafting. Lancet 1: 551.

Ciba Foundation Symposium (1973) Corneal Graft Failure, p. 344. Associated Scientific Publishers, Amsterdam/London/New York.

Ehlers N. and Ahrons S. (1971) Corneal transplantation and histocompatibility. Acta Ophthalmol. (Kbh) 49: 513.

Ehlers N. and Kissmeyer-Nielsen F. (1973) Influence of histocompatiblity on the fate of the corneal transplant. In: Corneal Graft Failure, Ciba Foundation Symposium 15: 307. Associated Scientific Publishers, Amsterdam/London/New York.

Ehlers N. and Kissmeyer-Nielsen F. (1979) Corneal transplantation and HLA-compatibility. Acta Ophthalmol. (Kbh) 57: 738-741.

Gibbs D.C., Batchelor J.R., Werb A., Schlesinger W. and Casey T.A. (1974) The influence of tissue-type compatibility on the fate of full-thickness corneal grafts. Trans. Ophthalmol. Soc. UK 94: 101.

Gibbs D.C., Batchelor J.R., Casey T.A., Werb, A. Liakos G. and Taylor C. (1979) HLA-matching and corneal graft rejection. Doc. Ophthalmol. Proc. Ser. 20: 139-149.

Khodadoust A.A. (1973) The allograft rejection reaction: the leading cause of late failure of clinical corneal grafts. In: Corneal Graft Failure. Ciba Foundation Symposium 15: 151. Associated Scientific Publishers, Amsterdam/London/New York.

Khodadoust A.A. and Abizedeh A. (1979) The fate of corneal regrafts after previous rejection reactions. Doc. Ophthalmol. Proc. Ser. 20: 115-122.

Kok-van Alphen C.C. (1954) Bijdrage tot de keratoplastiek. Diss. Eduard IJdo, Leiden.

Kok-van Alphen C.C. and Völker-Dieben H.J. (1979) Diagnosis and treatment of complications in the follow-up period after corneal transplantation.

Maumenee A.E. (1951) The influence of donor-recipient sensitization on corneal grafts. Am.J.Ophthalmol. 34: 142.

Paufique M. (1948) Les greffes de la cornée, pp. 134-136. Masson, Paris.

Peto R., Pike M.C., Armitage P., Breslow N.E., Cox D.R., Howard S.V., Mantel N. McPherson K., Peto J. and Smith P.G. (1976) Design and analysis of randomized clinical trials requiring prolonged observation of each patient. I.Br.J.Cancer 34: 585.

Van Rood J.J. (1979) Microlymphocytotoxicity method. In: NIAID Manual of tissue typing techniques (Ed.: J. Ray) National Institutes of Health (NIH) (80-545) Maryland, U.S.A.: 104.

Stark W.J., Taylor H.R. and Bias W.B. (1979) Keratoplasty and transplantation antigens. Doc. Ophthalmol. Proc. Ser. 20: 123-130.
Vannas S. (1970) Some features of ophthalmology in Finland. Am.J.Ophthalmol. 70: 422-426.
Vannas S., Karjalainen P., Ruusuvaara A. and Tiilikainen A. (1976) HLA-compatible donor for prevention of allograft reaction. Albrecht von Grafes Arch. Klin. Ophthalmol. 198: 217.
Völker-Dieben H.J., Kok-van Alphen C.C., Oosterhuis J.A., van Dorp G. and van Leeuwen A. (1977) First experiences with HLA-matched corneal grafts in high risk cases. Doc. Ophthalmol. 44: 39-48.
Völker-Dieben H.J., Kok-van Alphen C.C., Kruit P.J. (1978) Advances and disappointments, indications and restrictions regarding HLA-matched corneal grafts in high risk cases. Doc. Ophthalmol. 46: 219-22

CHAPTER 7

The interactions of HLA-DR, donor graft size and corneal vascularisation of the recipient on graft survival*

Summary

This is the first report on the effect of HLA-DR matching on corneal graft survival in which 79 HLA-A, -B and -DR typed donor recipient pairs were studied, with a follow-up period ranging from 3 months to 3 years. Neither in the total group of 79 cases nor in a subgroup of 57 vascularized recipient corneas a significant effect of the number of HLA-DR mismatches was observed. HLA-DR antigenic material was demonstrated only at a distance of 3.5 to 4.0 mm from the center of the cornea. Analyses of the influence of corneal graft diameter in 821 grafts revealed a highly significant inverse correlation between graft diameter and corneal graft survival ($p=0.00005$). This inverse correlation remained significant when only 510 first grafts were analyzed ($p=0.023$). The same inverse correlation was observed in 311 moderately or severely vascularized corneas ($p=0.0003$) as well as in a subgroup of 161 first grafts in moderately or severely vascularized corneas ($p=0.017$). An analysis of the influence of corneal graft diameter of 147 grafts in donor-recipient pairs with less than 3 HLA-A and -B mismatches revealed no significant influence of graft size ($p=0.062$); however, a subgroup of 130 moderately or severely vascularized corneas demonstrated, again, a significant difference in graft survival between small and large grafts ($p=0.03$). We suggest that the restricted distribution of HLA antigens is the main cause for the absence of influence of HLA-DR matching whose effects can probably only be observed in vascularized corneas with large grafts.

Introduction

When Paufique described in 1948 the 'Maladie du Greffon', at that time an unexplained allergic phenomenon, it was in fact the first description of the clinical picture of corneal graft rejection. Since then, knowledge of the mechanism responsible for the destruction of corneal grafts has increased and the possibility that corneal graft rejection may be due to immunological factors became accepted in the early seventies (Ehlers and Ahrons, 1971).

In previous studies, we were able to demonstrate the beneficial influence of prospective HLA-A and -B matching on corneal graft survival (chapter 6 and 10). Since it has been reported that HLA-DR matching has a beneficial effect on kidney graft survival (Persijn et al. 1978, Moen et al. 1980, Ting and Morris 1980), we were interested in studying the effect of HLA-DR matching on the survival of corneal grafts.

Although the HLA-A, -B and -C antigens are present on almost all cells,

* *For colour plates, see pp. 72ff.*

the DR locus antigens have been found only on a limited number of cell types in the eye. These antigens are known to be present on dendritic cells (Langerhans cells) in the corneal epithelium and have also been reported in the substantia propria towards the periphery of the cornea and on conjunctival epithelium (Braude and Chandler 1983).

Materials and methods

From January 1976 to January 1983, 858 full thickness keratoplasties were performed. All grafts were performed by only one of two surgeons (Völker-Dieben and Kok-van Alphen). Of these keratoplasties, 281 were performed in HLA-A and -B typed donor-recipient pairs. Seventy nine cornea donors were typed for HLA-DR. Their recipients were typed for HLA-DR retrospectively. No prospective selection for HLA-DR matching was performed. Blood grouping and all HLA-A, -B, -C and -DR typings of the patients and donors were performed in the National Reference Center, Leyden (Department of Immunohaematology, University Hospital). The methods used are described in a previous article (Van Rood et al. 1976) and in chapter 5.

All patients and graft donors were of Dutch Caucasoid origin. All survival times were calculated using the actuarial life table method. The significance of the differences between the various classes were tested with a X^2 statistic derived from the logrank test (Peto et al. 1976). The numbers to the right of the follow-up curves indicate the numbers of the patients at risk at the start of the study (fig. 1-3). The criterium for graft survival for corneal allografts is as described by Jones (1973) with the clarity of the cornea as the major criterium.

Results

Seventy nine keratoplasties were performed with HLA-A, -B, -C and -DR typed donor material. The survival of those grafts did not differ significantly from the remaining 779 grafts, nor from the remaining 107 HLA-A and -B matched corneal grafts (figures not shown).

As shown in table 1, the number of HLA-DR mismatches did not significantly influence the graft survival of these 79 grafts. No exclusions for whatever reason had been made. The one, two and three years graft survival was 100% for the group of 6 grafts with zero DR mismatches, for the group of 41 grafts with one DR mismatch 86.5%, 80.7% and 80.7% respectively while the group of 32 grafts with two DR mismatches demonstrated a corneal graft survival of 90.0% at one, two and three years.

Since the influence of HLA-A and -B matching was only significant in

Table 1. The effect of HLA-DR mismatches on 79 corneal grafts

DR mismatches	N	Actuarial survival at 1 year	2 years	3 years
0	6	100.0	100.0	100.0
1	41	86.5	80.7	80.7
2	32	90.0	90.0	90.0

$X^2 = 1.27$; $p = 0.53$

vascularized corneas (chapter 6), we made a subdivision according the degree of corneal vascularisation in the group of 79 DR matched grafts. Fifty seven recipient corneas were moderately or severely vascularized, while 22 corneas were only slightly vascularized or did not show any vessel ingrowth. No significant influence of DR matching was observed in the total of 79 cases nor in the 57 vascularized corneas (table 2).

Table 2. The effect of HLA-DR mismatches in 57 corneal grafts performed in moderately or severely vascularized corneas

DR mismatches	N	Actuarial survival at 1 year	2 years	3 years
0	5	100.0	100.0	100.0
1	28	84.3	74.9	74.9
2	24	87.1	87.1	87.1

$X^2 = 1.26$; $p = 0.53$

The effect of HLA-A and -B mismatches was examined in the three groups of corneal grafts with zero, one or two DR mismatches (table 3). There were no significant differences in the distribution of HLA-A and -B mismatches in the different HLA-DR mismatched groups.

All 9 graft failures, 8 irreversible (immunological) rejections and 1 non-immunological failure were observed in the group of vascularized corneas. The 8 immunological graft failures in vascularized grafts did not correlate significantly with the number of HLA-DR mismatches.

Table 3. Distribution of HLA-A and -B mismatches in the three HLA-DR mismatch classes

DR mismatches	HLA-A and -B mismatches 0	1	2	3	4	Total
0	0	2	4	0	0	6
1	4	13	11	8	5	41
2	4	9	11	7	1	32
Total	8	24	26	15	6	79

$X^2 = 7.17$; $p = 0.52$ NS

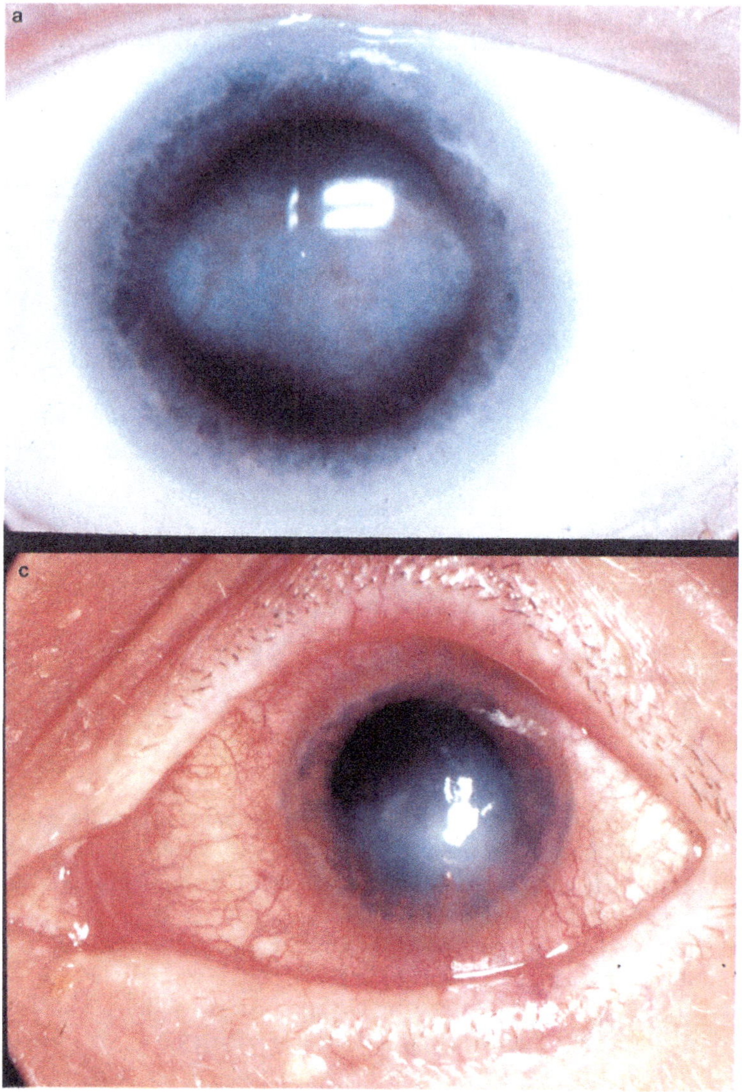

Colour plate 1: Examples of the 4 levels of corneal vascularisation.

a. Non: No vessel ingrowth.
c. Moderate: Vessel ingrowth in more than one quadrant.

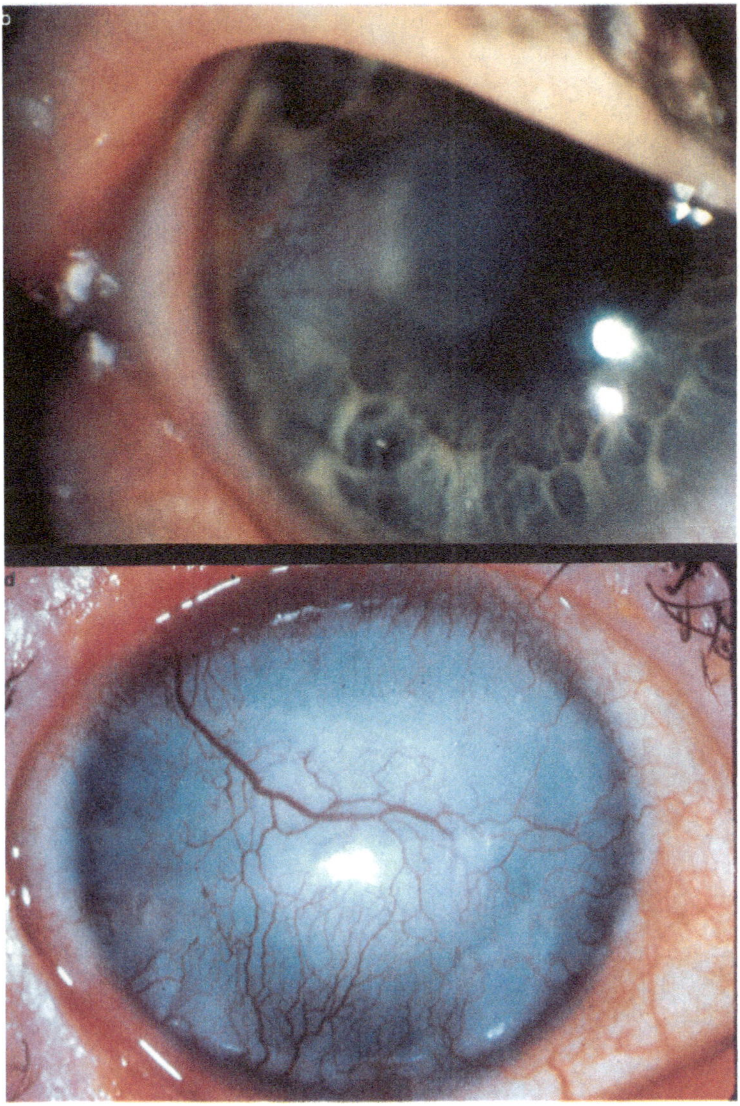

b. Slight: Vessel ingrowth in only one quadrant.
d. Severe: Vessel ingrowth in all four quadrants and in the centre of the cornea.

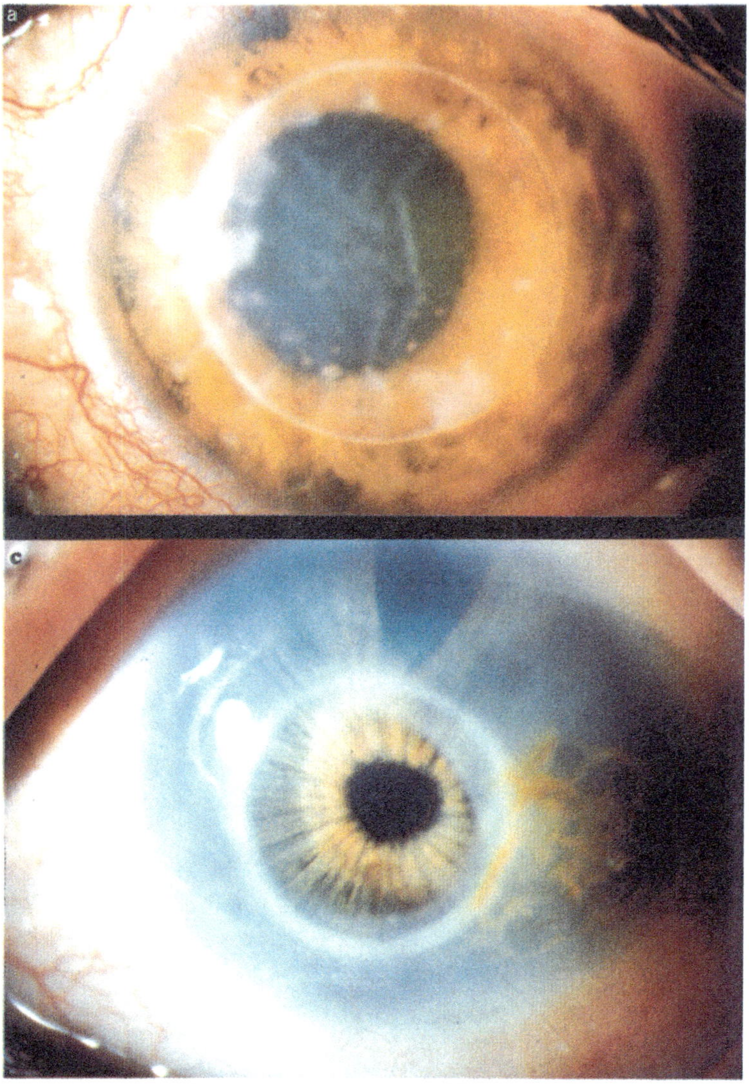

Colour plate 2

a. Rate corneal graft rejection, 21 months after grafting. Oedema of the graft with signs of inflammation in the anterior segment including ciliary flush and cells and usually a slight flare in the anterior chamber.
c. Small corneal graft,28 years after transplantatio; graft diameter is 6.0 mm.

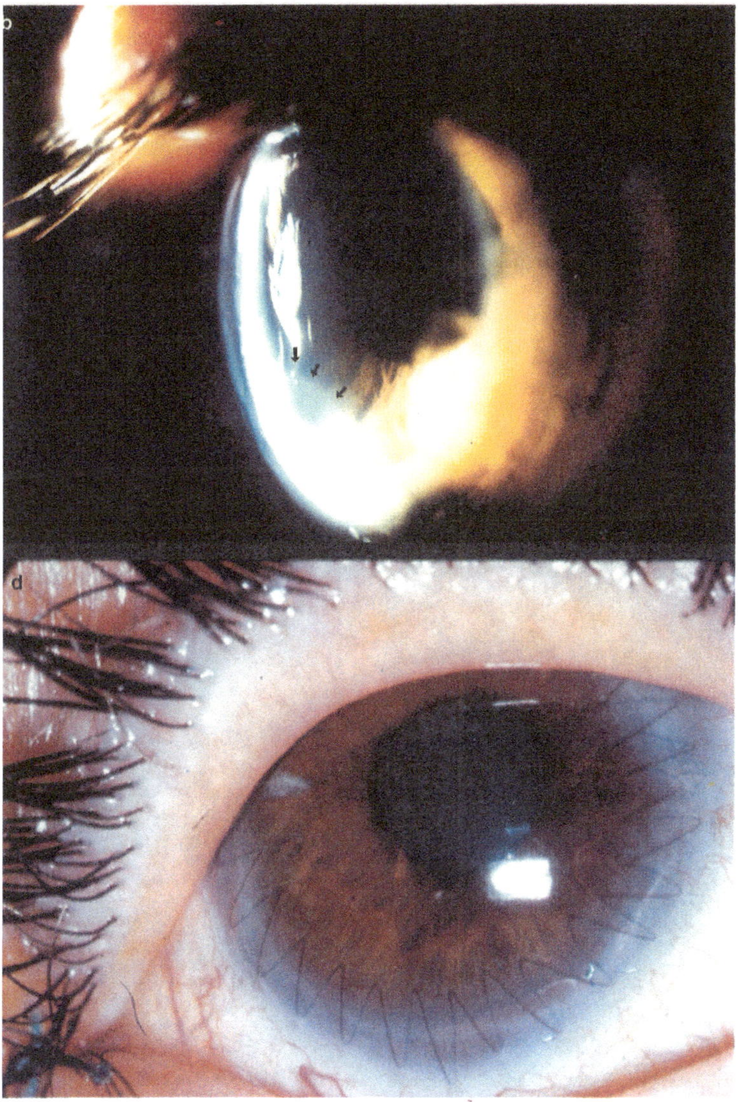

b. Corneal graft rejection, 7 weeks after grafting.
d. Large corneal graft, 7 months after transplantation; graft diameter is 9.0 mm.

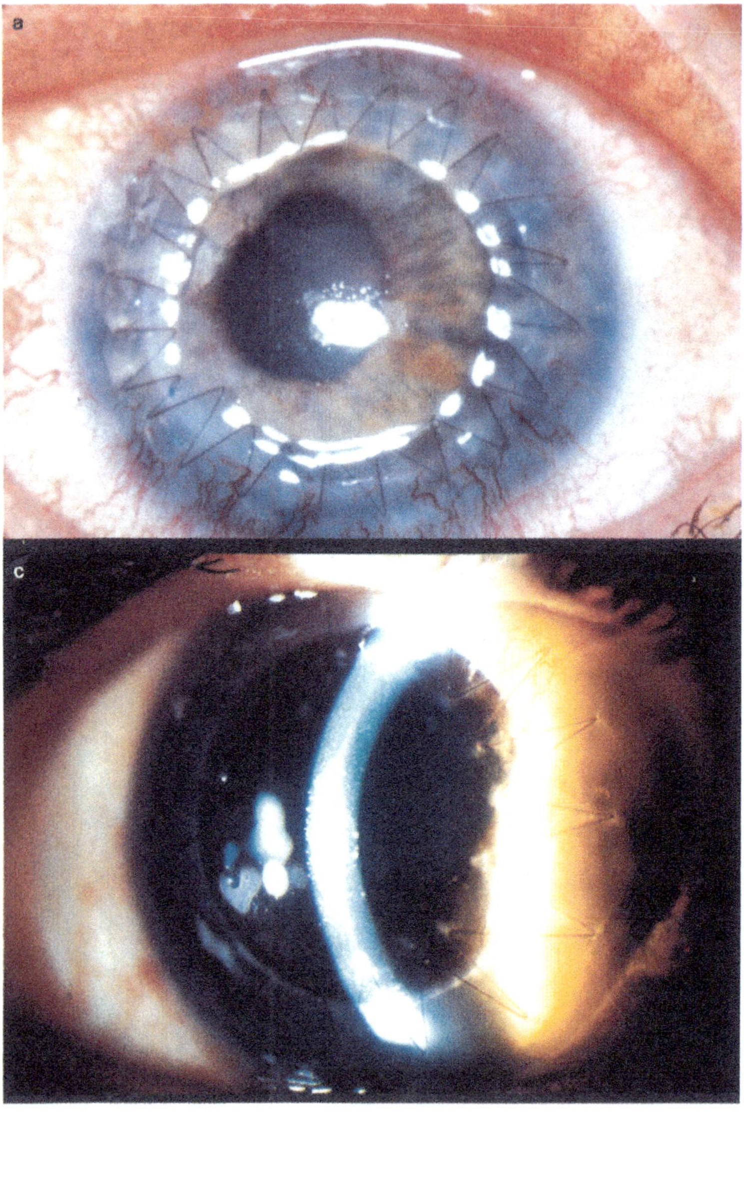

Colour plate 3

a. Clear corneal graft, 4 weeks after transplantation in a 5-year-old girl. The initial disease was recurrent herpes keratitis.
c. In severely vascularized eyes, small white spots were observed where the suture penetrates the recipient and/or the donor cornea.

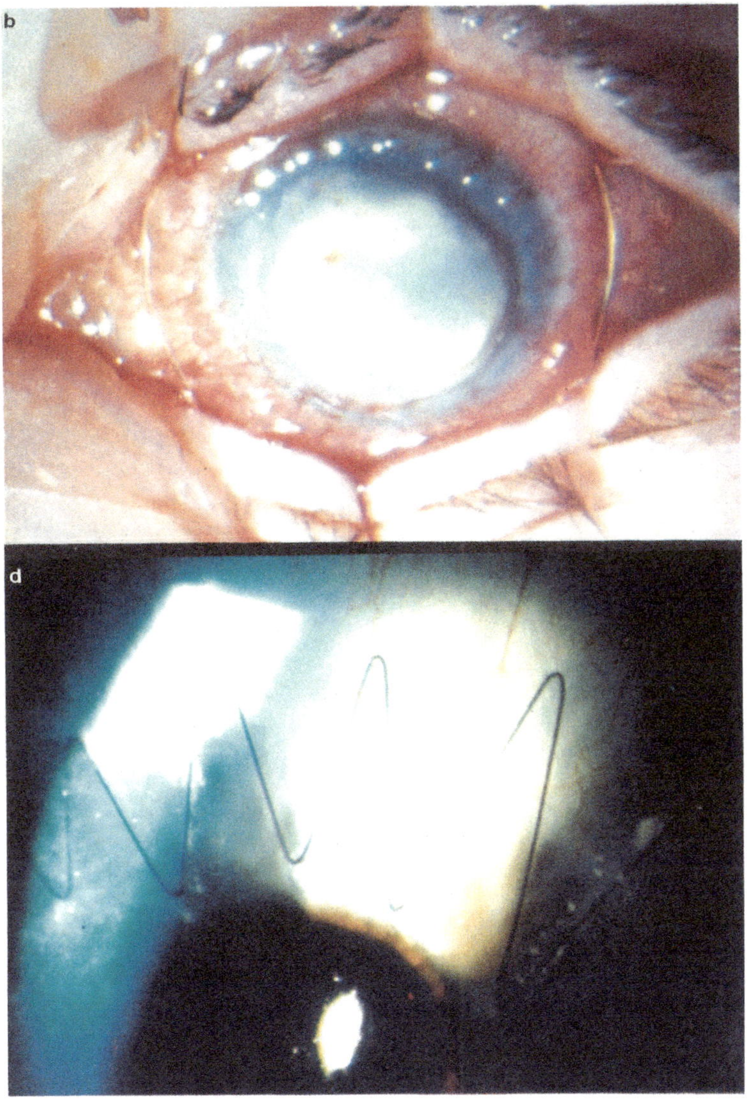

b. Pseudomonas infection 5 months later. This cornea was regrafted *à chaud* due to lysis of the graft.
d. In this enlargement the white spots also appear along the length of the suture.

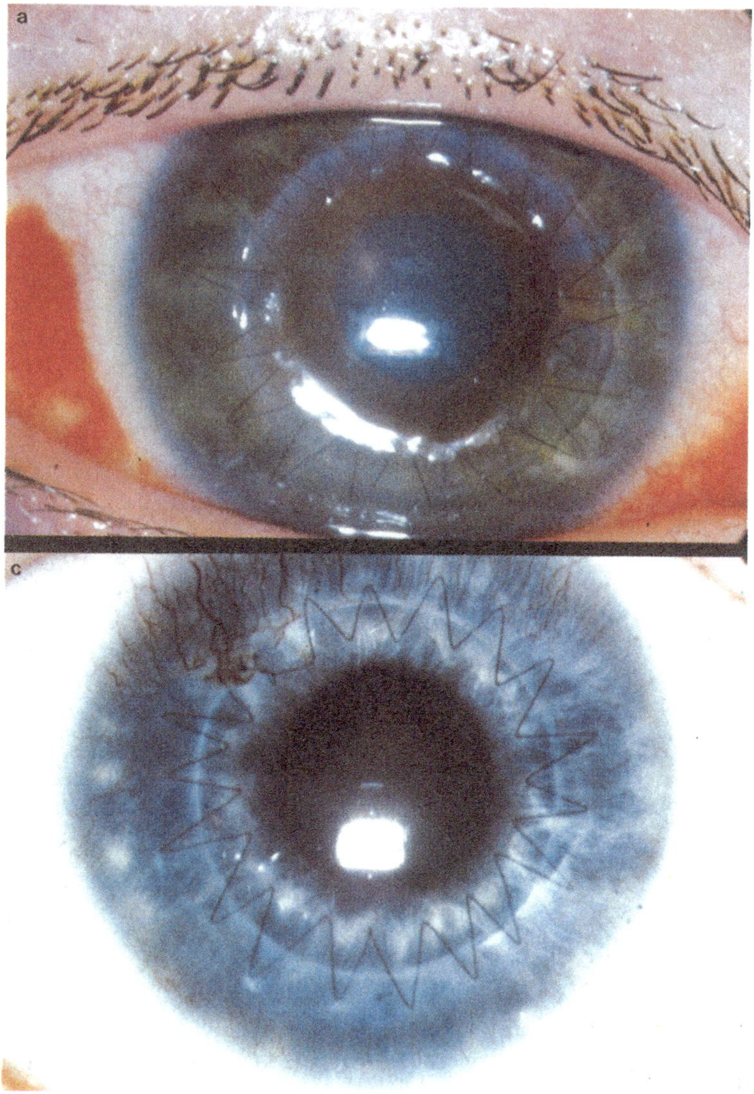

Colour plate 4

a. Clear corneal graft, 4 months later transplantation in a 7-year-old boy. The initial disease was recurrent herpes keratitis.
c. Clear corneal graft 4 months after transplantation; visual acuity 0.6 with correction.

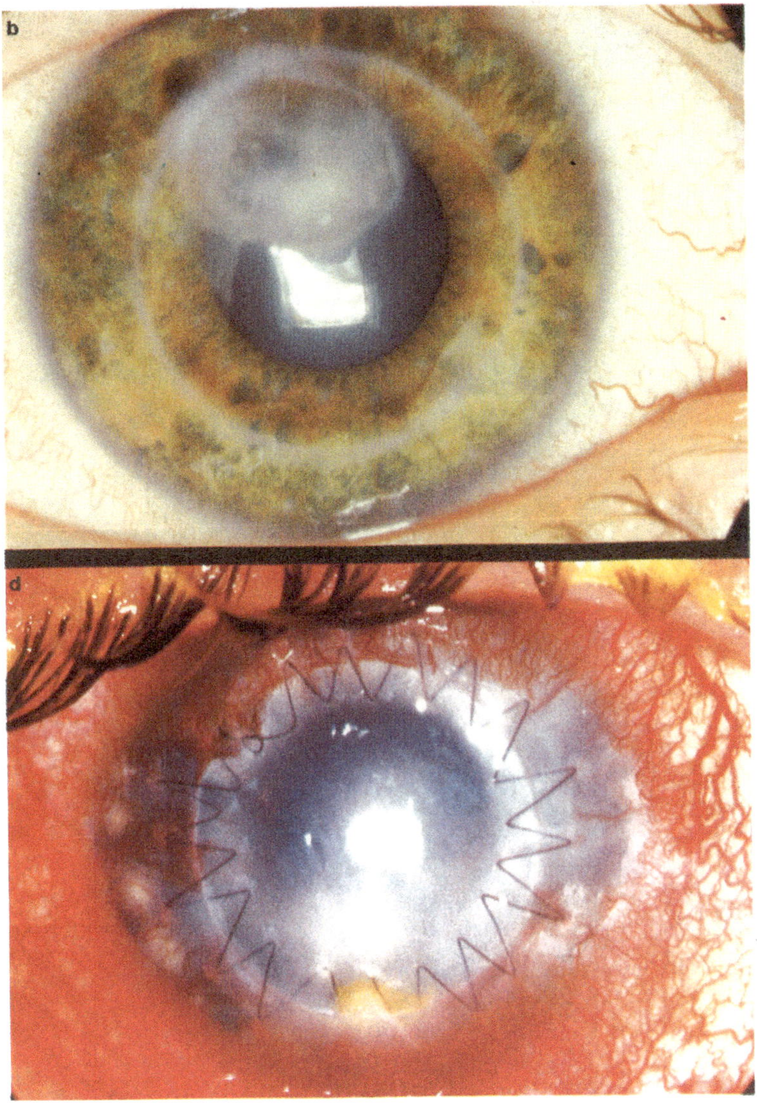

b. Pneumococcal ulcer, 7 months after grafting.
d. The same graft 2 weeks later. A severe graft rejection destroyed the restored visual acuity.

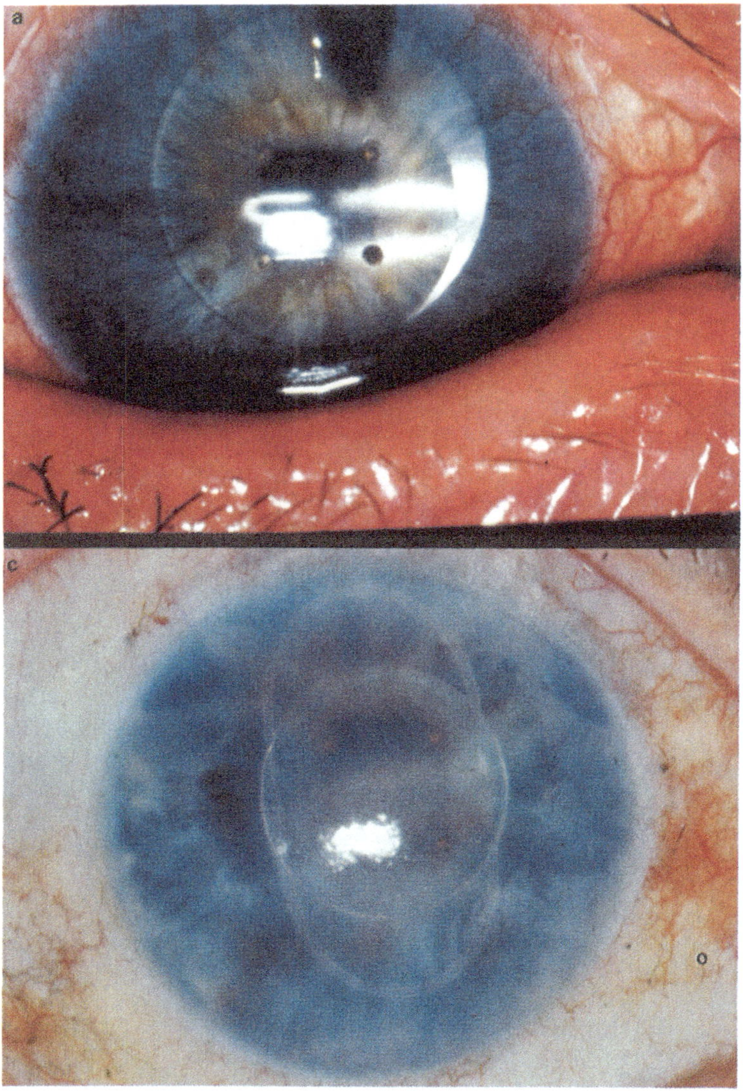

Colour plate 5

a. Pseudophakic eye with a platinum safety pin medallion, 1 year after cataract surgery; visual acui 0.6 with correction.
c. Secondary endothelial decompensation 4 years after intracapsular cataract extraction and inse tion of a 4 loop Binkhorst lens.

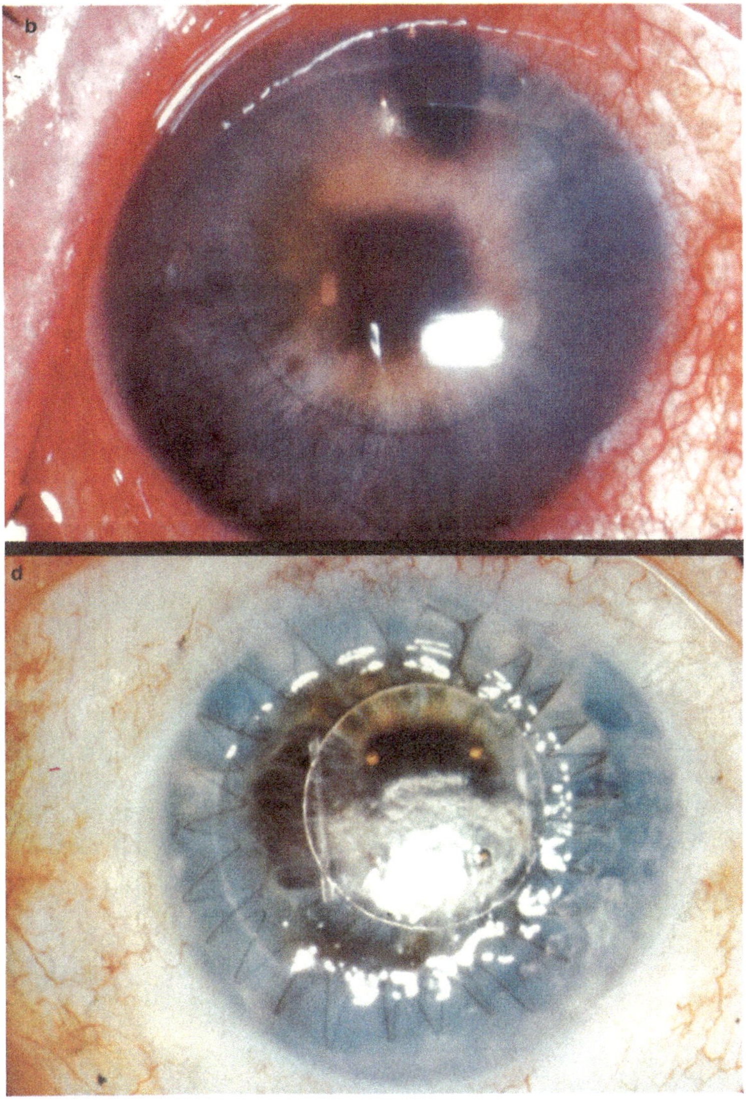

b. Thirty-two months later, the patient was referred for a penetrating keratoplasty because of secondary endothelial decompensation.
d. The anterior loops of this lens were cut off during keratoplasty.

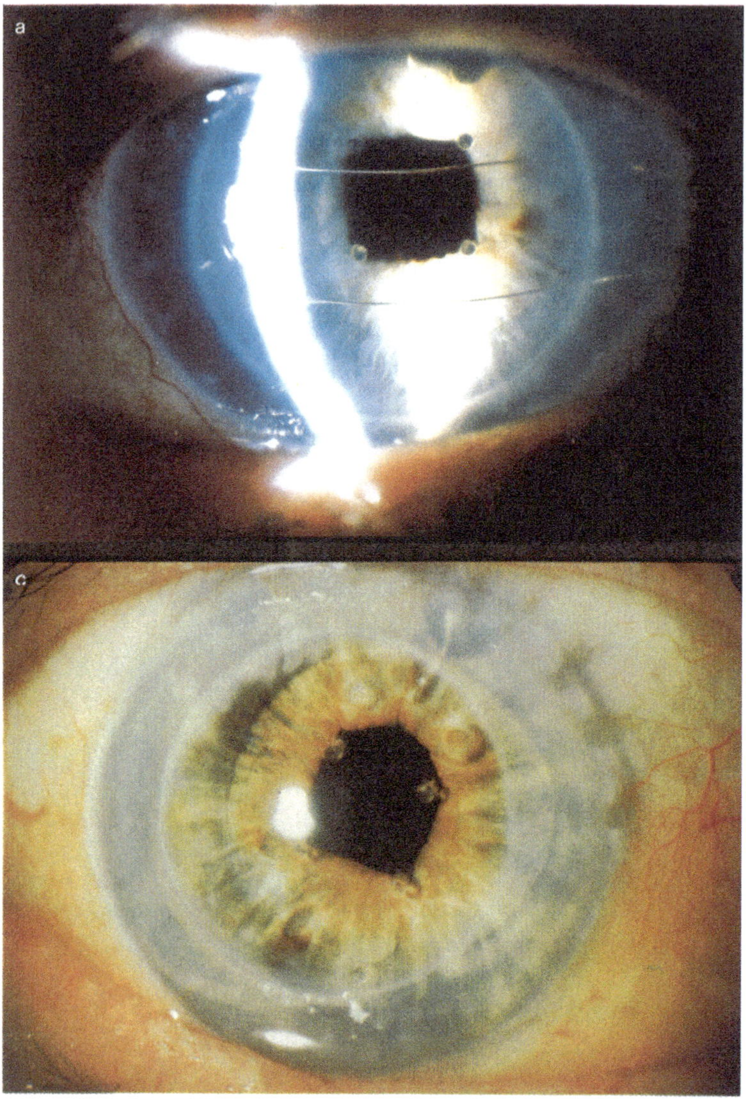

Colour plate 6

a. In this case with marked pseudophakodonesis combined with secondary endothelial decompensation, the intra-ocular lens has been stabilized before corneal transplantation with two stainless steel sutures.
c. Although the anterior synechiae between the intra-ocular lens and the cornea were separated during keratoplasty they tend to reoccur in the post-operative period.

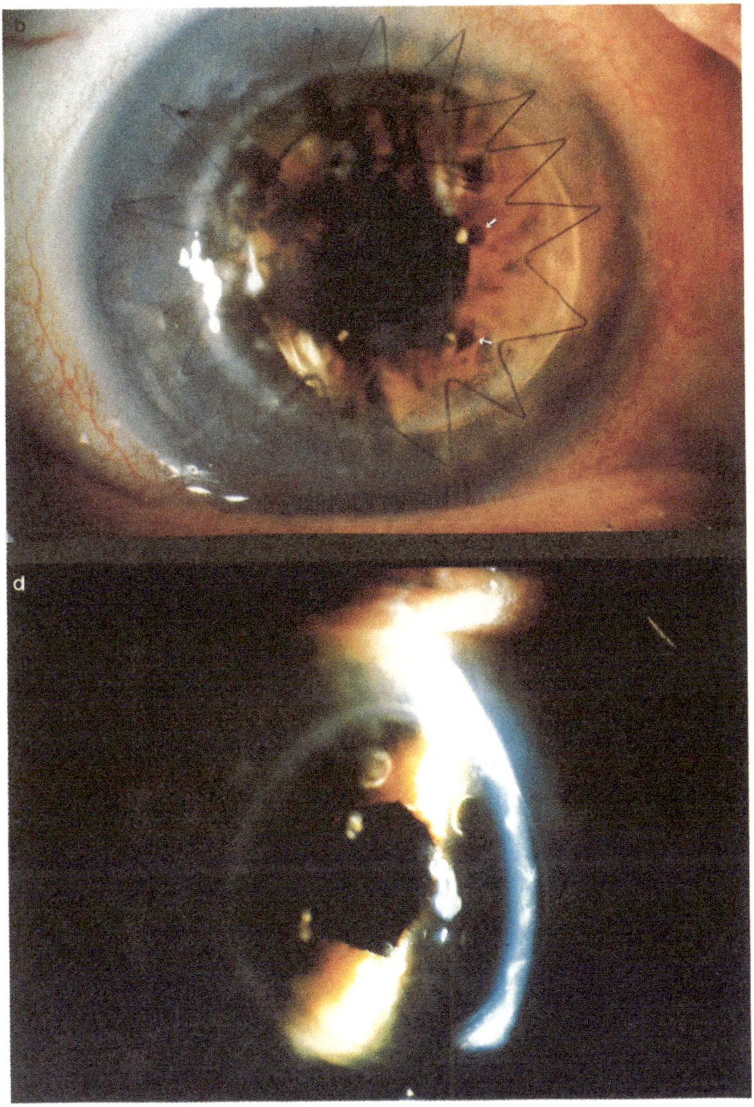

b. Tilted intra-ocular lens. The shadows of the fixation points of the nasal loop (white arrows) indicate that the lens is markedly displaced above the irisplane.

d. A renewed contact between lens and cornea at the 12 o'clock position occurred five months postoperatively

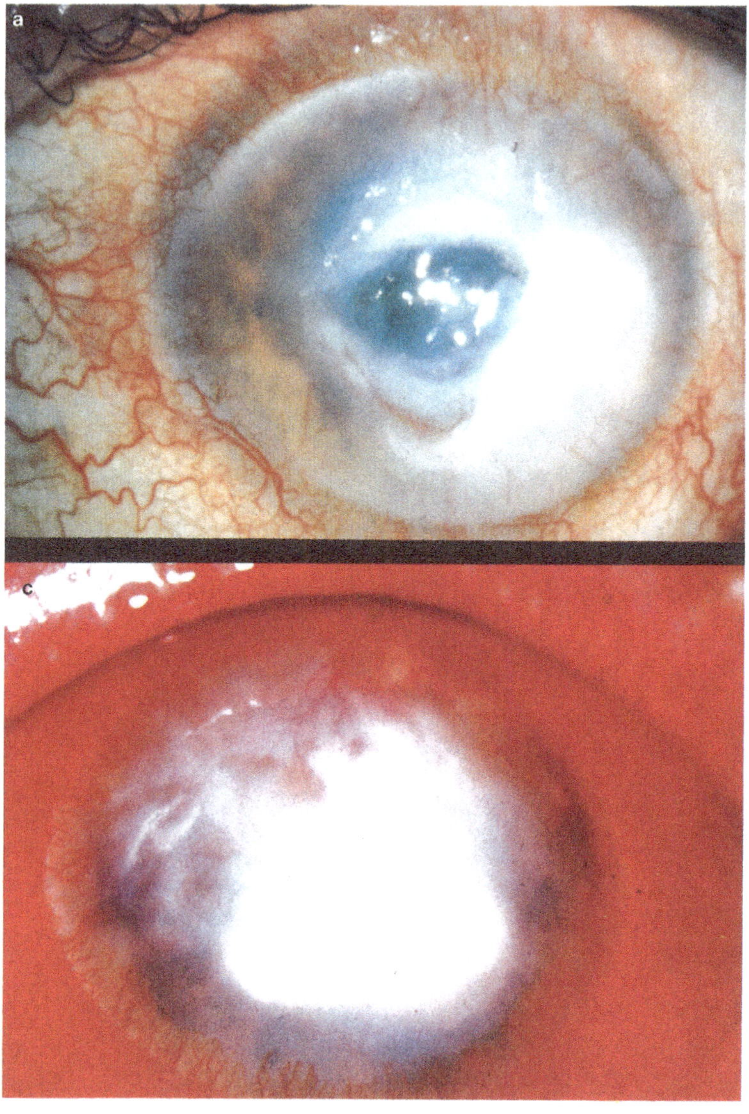

Colour plate 7

a. and b. Corneal graft, 13 months post-operatively (b) performed *à chaud* because of a descemetocule (a).

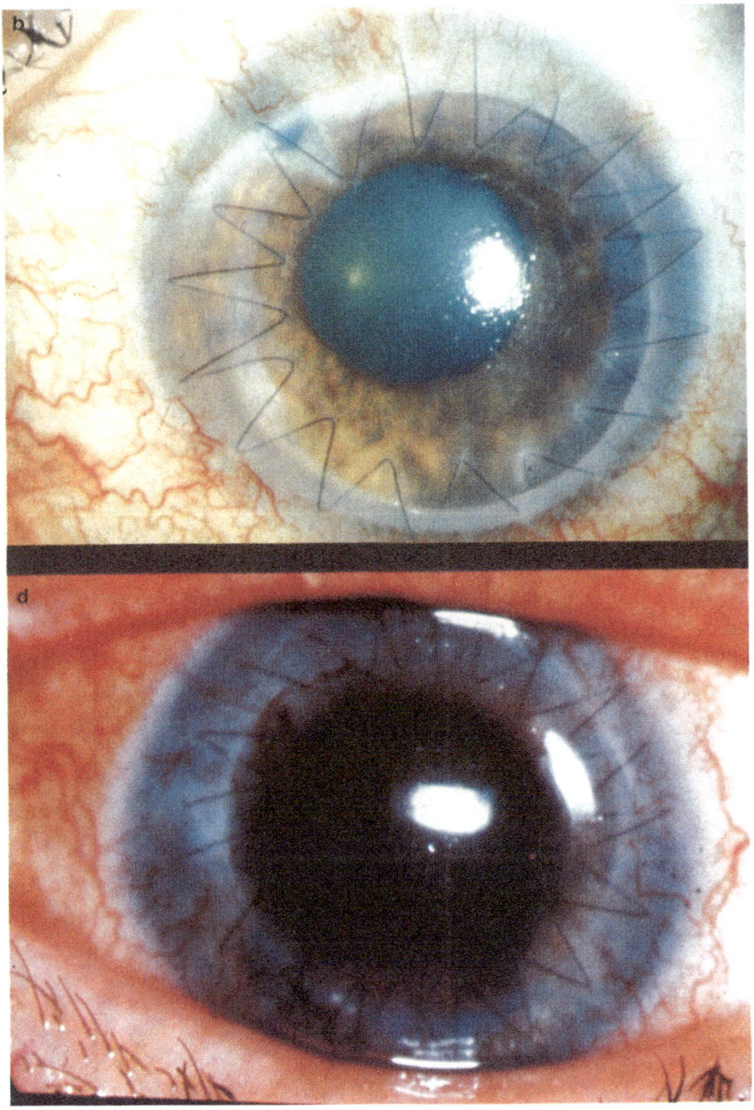

c. and d. Corneal graft, 11 months post-operatively (b) performed *à chaud* because of constant severe herpes keratitis (a).

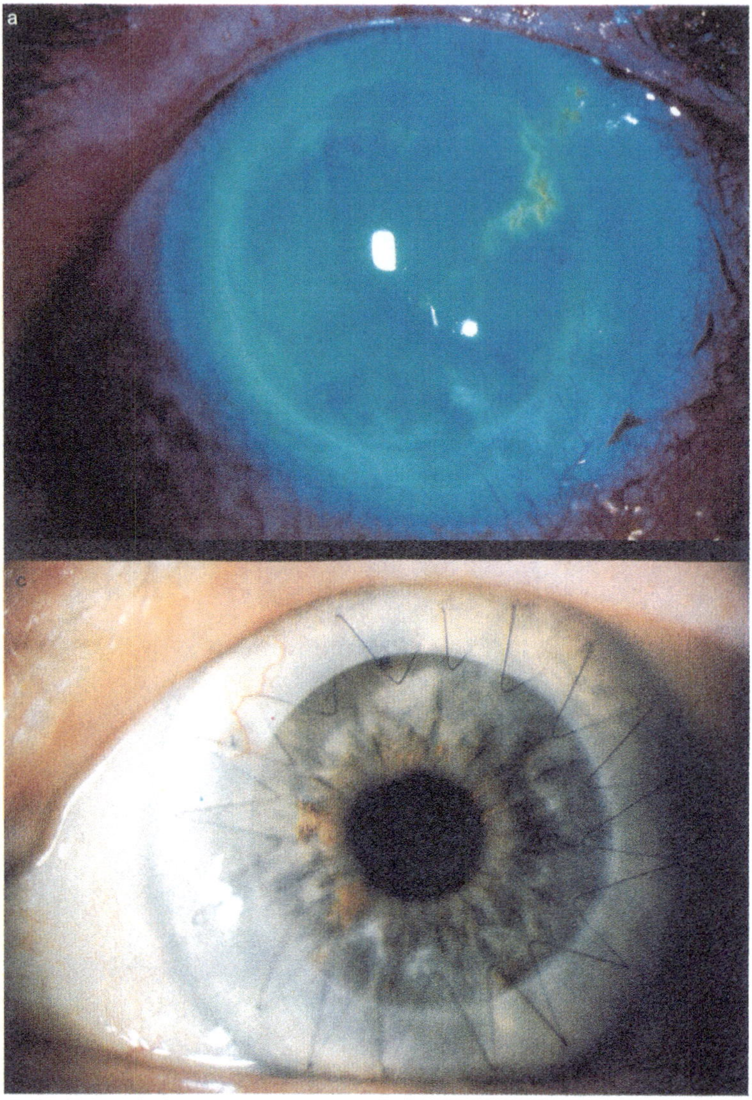

Colour plate 8
a. Recurrence of herpes simplex infection in a graft along the path of nerve ingrowth, 28 months after transplantation.
c. Attraction of vascular ingrowth by a long suture knot.

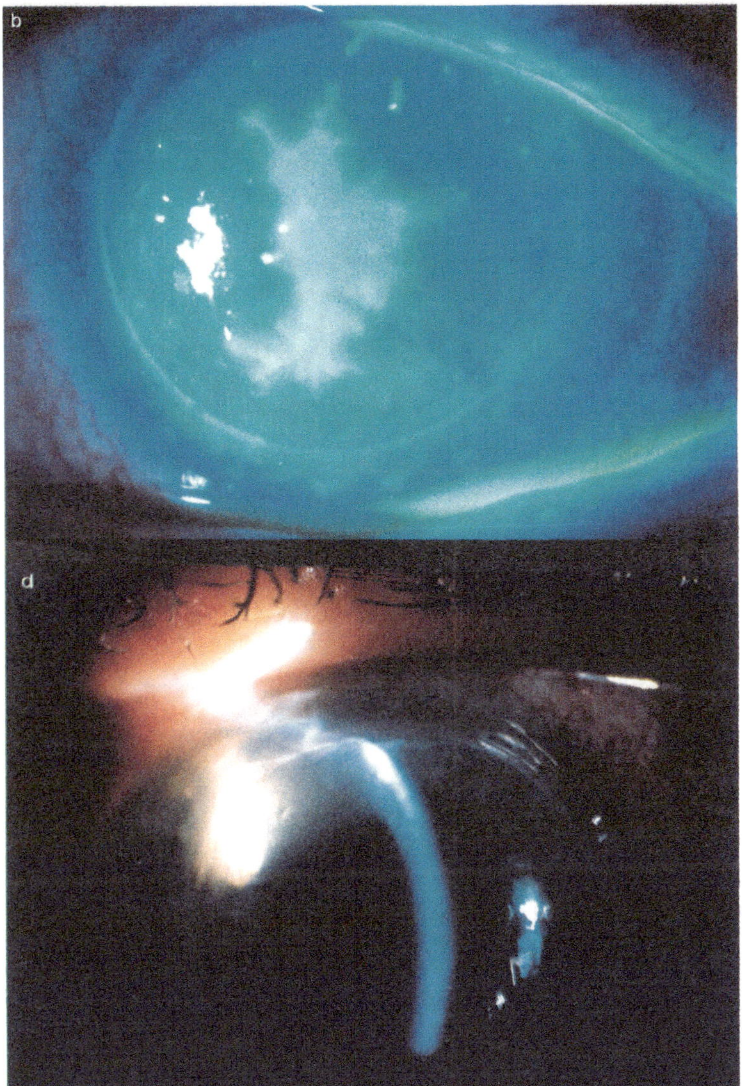

b. Geographic ulcer resulting from a failure to treat a recurrent herpes infection.
d. Local graft rejection, possibly induced by such a knot, suggests that they should be removed.

Since Mayer et al. (1983) and Rodriques (1981) demonstrated the presence of HLA-DR antigens only in the peripheral one third of the cornea, we decided to classify all our cases into three groups according to the size of their donor corneal buttons. In group 1, small grafts, the diameter of the donor button is 7.1 mm or less. These small donor buttons are most probably negative for HLA-DR. In group 2, medium sizedgrafts, the diameter of these donor buttons ranged from 7.2 mm to 7.9 mm. In group 3, large grafts, the diameter of the donor buttons is 8.0 mm or more. These large donor buttons are most probably positive for HLA-DR. The diameters were recorded of 821 donor buttons; 194 were in group 1 (small), 328 were in group 2 (medium) and the remaining 289 in group 3 (large) (See colour plate 2, c and d).

There was a highly significant (p=0.00005) inverse correlation between graft diameter and corneal graft survival (fig. 1A). The percentage of corneal

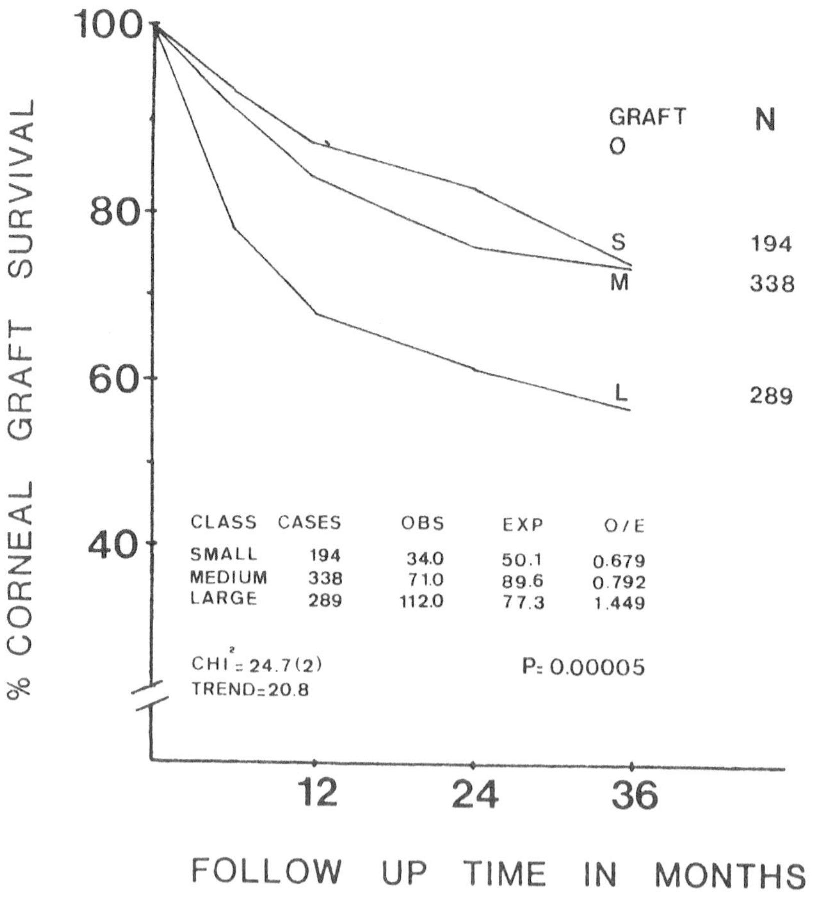

Figure 1A. The effect of graft diameter on corneal graft survival (N=821).

graft survival for the small grafts was 87.3%, 83.6% and 72.3%, for the medium sized grafts 84.4%, 76.3% and 72.2% while for the large grafts it was 68.9%, 61.1% and 57.1% at one, two and three years.

We repeated the analysis using only first grafts (N=510) in order to avoid the effect of presensitization by prior graft failures. In chapter 5 we have reported that the influence of pregnancies and/or pretransplant blood transfusions on corneal graft survival was not significant. The effect of the graft diameter in these cases remained statistically significant (p=0.023) (fig. 1B). The graft survival was, for the smaller grafts 88.0%, 83.3% and 76.3%, for the medium sized grafts 83.0%, 76.8% and 73.4% and for the large grafts 76.4%, 70.8% and 67.2% at one, two and three years. The ranking of

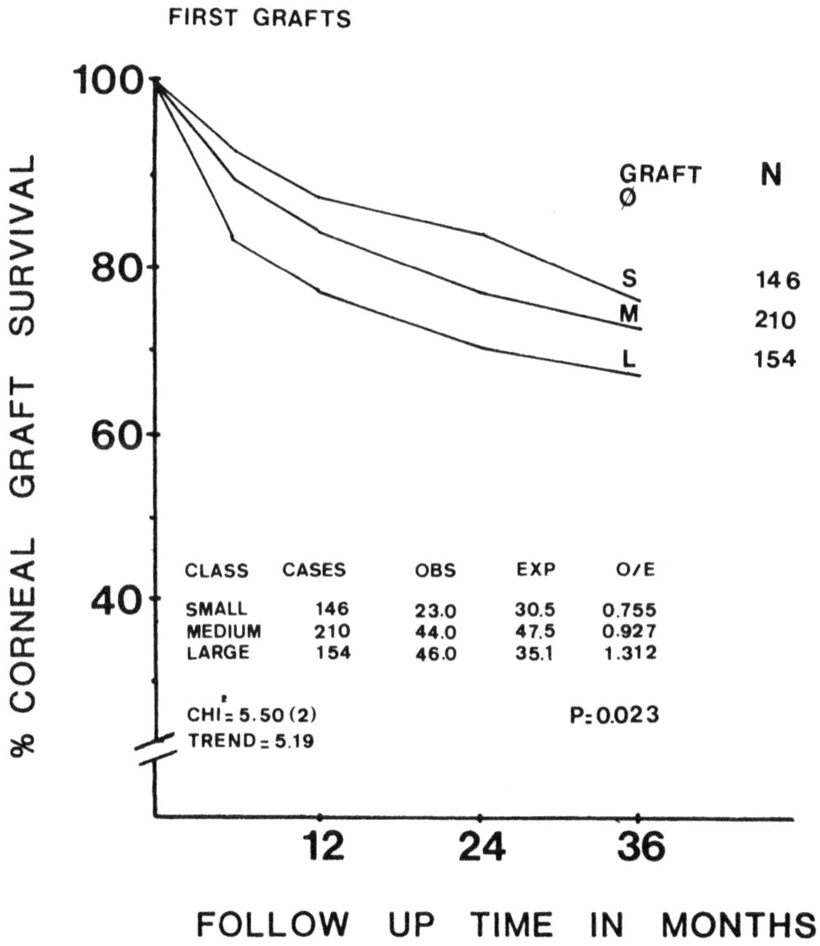

Figure 1B. The effect of graft diameter on corneal graft survival in first grafts (N=510).

the survival curves of the three classes was the same as in the total analysis (see fig. 1A).

Since the effect of HLA-A and -B matching was statistically significant only in vascularized corneas (chapter 5), we examined the combined effect of donor button size and the degree of vascularisation of the recipient cornea. In non or slightly vascularized corneas, the percentage of clear corneas was not significantly different when the group of small donor buttons was compared to the group of large ones (84.4% and 80.5% survival at 3 years, for small and large grafts respectively) (curves not shown). There was also no significant difference when only first grafts were examined (81.2% and 80.5% survival at 3 years for small and large grafts respectively) (curves not shown). Note that in the latter cases the survival of the smaller grafts was slightly better than of the larger grafts.

In contrast to the non or slightly vascularized group, we observed in the moderately or severely vascularized corneas, a highly significant difference in graft survival for these two donor button size categories (p=0.0003) (fig. 2A).

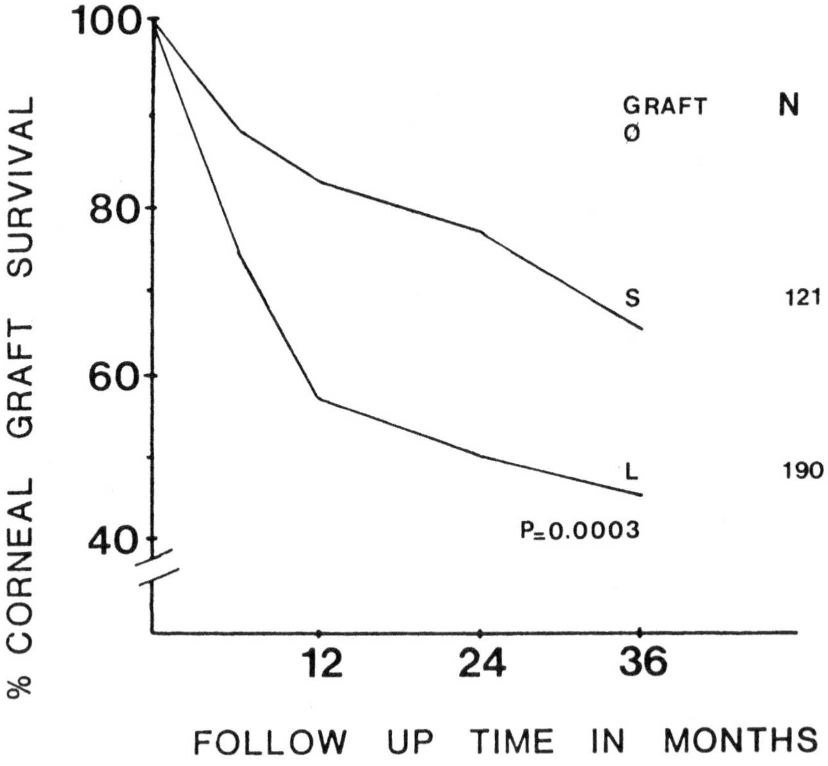

Figure 2A. The effect of graft diameter on corneal graft survival in moderately or severely vascularised corneas (N=311) (S = small, L = large).

The small grafts demonstrated a graft survival of 82.7%, 78.2% and 64.8% while only 58.7%, 50.0% and 44.6% of the group of large grafts were clear at one, two and three years. In an analysis of only first grafts in vascularized corneas, the effect of donor button size on graft survival remained significant (p=0.017) (fig. 2B). 83.3%, 77.2% and 71.9% clear grafts for the small donor buttons versus 64.9%, 58.4% and 53.0% for the larger buttons at one, two and three years.

An analysis of 147 donor-recipient pairs with less than 3 HLA-A and -B mismatches, of which 56 were small grafts versus 91 larger ones, revealed no significant influence of donor button size (fig. 3A) 85.1%, 85.1% and 68.6% clear grafts for the small donor buttons versus 70.5%, 60.6% and 57.4% for the larger buttons at one, two and three years. Examination of the survival of the 130 moderately or severely vascularized corneas within that group demonstrated a significant difference in graft survival between small and

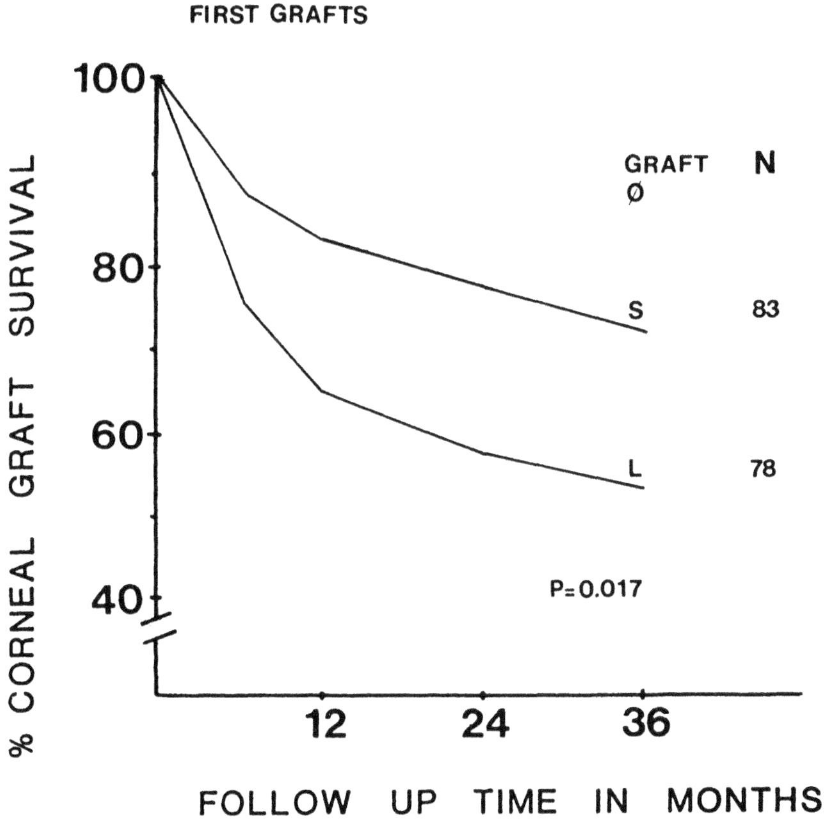

Figure 2B. The effect of graft diameter on corneal graft survival in moderately or severely vascularised corneas, first grafts only (N=161) (S = small, L = large).

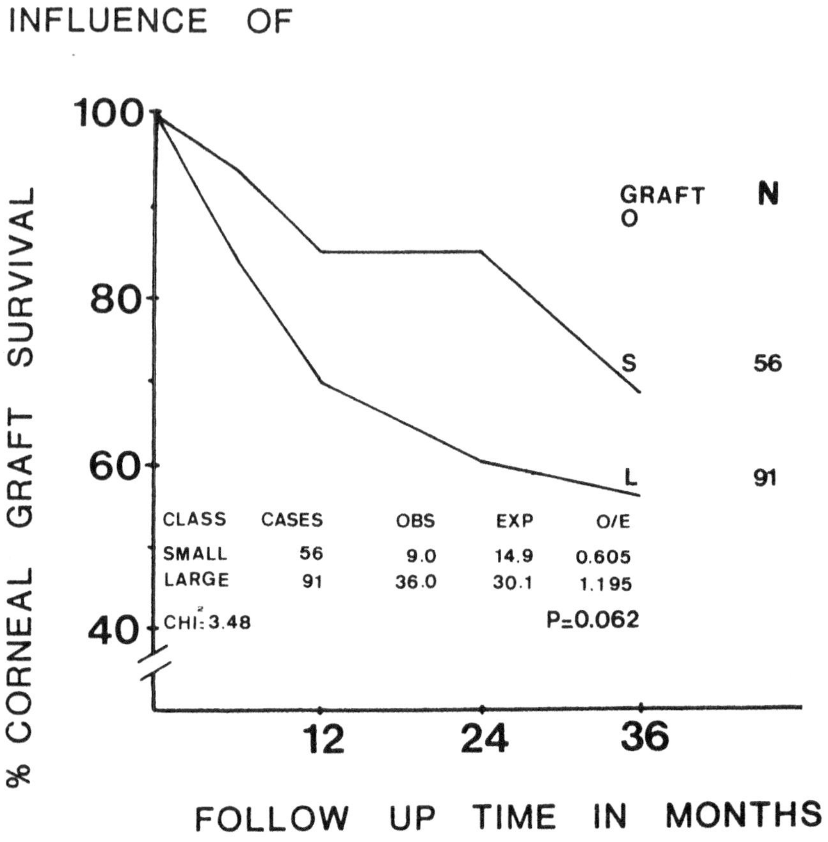

Figure 3A. The effect of graft diameter on corneal graft survival in HLA-A and -B matched grafts, in donor-recipient pairs with less than 3 HLA-A and -B mismatches (N=147).

large grafts with a p value of 0.03 (fig. 3B): 86.6%, 86.6% and 67.3% clear grafts for the small donor buttons versus 66.9%, 55.7% and 52.2% for the larger buttons at one, two and three years. Although the difference in significance levels in figures 3A and 3B are relatively slight, there are still some intriguing differences between those two figures. The survival of the smaller donor corneas are very similar in the two analyses. Consequently, it is likely that the increased significance in fig. 3B was caused by a poorer survival of the larger donors corneas in recipients with vascularized corneas.

Discussion

The effect of HLA-DR matching on corneal graft survival has not yet been described. The importance of HLA-DR matching on kidney graft survival

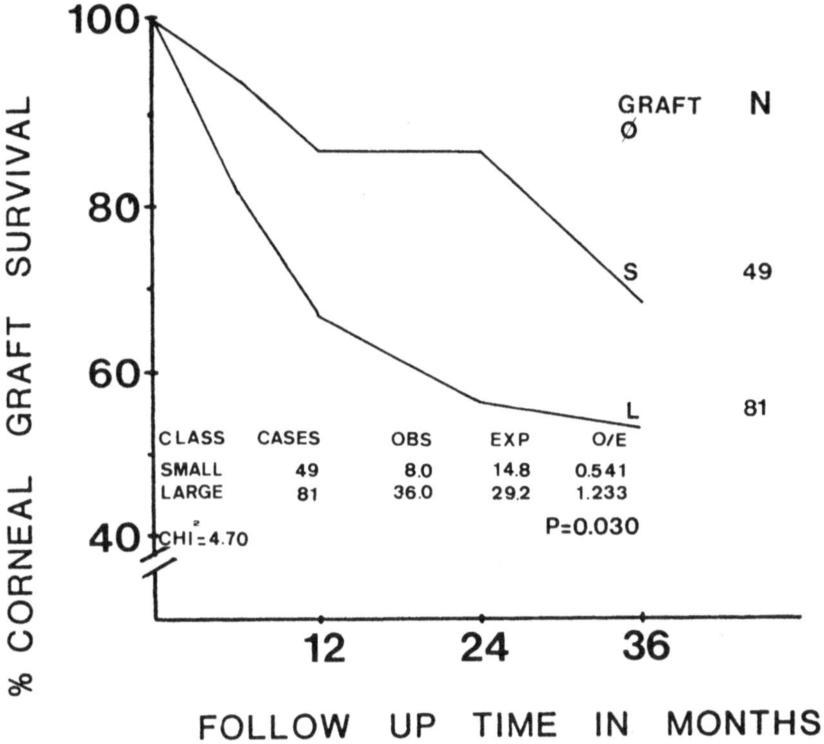

Figure 3B. The effect of graft diameter on corneal graft survival in HLA-A and -B matched grafts, donor-recipient pairs with less than 3 HLA-A and -B mismatches, in moderately or several vascularised corneas (N=130).

has been reported by several authors (Persijn et al. 1978, Moen et al. 1980, Ting and Morris 1980). In 1980 Moen et al., in a single center study, reported that the influence of HLA-A and -B matching on kidney graft survival was 'clearly less than that of HLA-DR matching'. In contrast to the reports on the beneficial effect of HLA-DR matching on kidney graft survival, we could not demonstrate a significant effect of HLA-DR matching on the survival of corneal grafts, neither in the total of 79 HLA-DR typed donor-recipient pairs nor in a selection of 57 vascularized recipient corneas.

Moen (1980) also reported that mismatches for the HLA-A and -B antigens increased the detrimental effect of HLA-DR mismatching on kidney graft survival. We could not confirm his results in our cornea transplants since we observed no significant differences in the distribution of the numbers of HLA-A and -B mismatches in the different DR mismatch classes (see table 2 and 3).

During the period covered by this study, the epithelial layers of the donor corneas were not routinely removed before transplantation. Consequently, large donor buttons with a diameter greater than 7.9 mm could be expected to contain not only more HLA-DR antigenic material but also more HLA-A and -B antigenic material than the smaller buttons. The latter are reported to be non antigenic with respect to HLA-DR and contain only small amounts of HLA-A and -B antigenic material. We suggest that the restricted distribution of HLA-DR antigenic material in the cornea, i.e. the dendritic Langerhans cells, beginning only at a distance of 3.5 to 4.0 mm from the center, is the main cause for the lack of influence of HLA-DR matching on corneal graft survival. Only a very small number of the dendritic Langerhans cells are present in the peripheral third of the corneal epithelium, 15 to 20 cells/mm^2 (Rodriques et al. 1981). Therefore, it is possible that the ability of the donor dendritic cells to trigger T helper cells in the recipient might be inadequate, especially in small grafts. That possibility is supported by the observation of Lechler and Batchelor (1982) who demonstrated that a minimum number of dendritic cells, 1x104 to 5x104, was required to destroy kidney grafts in rats. Therefore, our demonstration of the significant influence of graft diameter on corneal graft survival (fig. 1 to 3) is in concordance with the above hypothesis. However, larger grafts contain not only dendritic cells but also an increased antigenic load of HLA-A and -B antigens. The effect of graft diameter on corneal graft survival is observed only when the recipient corneas are moderately or severely vascularized (fig. 3B). Since dendritic cells are observed especially in vascular structures, the number of dendritic cells in vascularized recipient corneas might be increased to such an extent that the chance of triggering T helper cells by the donor HLA-DR antigens is increased and, therefore, be responsible for the adverse effect on graft survival.

Conclusions

We were unable to demonstrate any significant influence of HLA-DR matching on corneal graft survival.

On the basis of our analysis of the influence of corneal graft diameter and reports on the distribution of DR antigenic material in the cornea, we suggest that the effect of DR matching on corneal graft survival can only be observed in vascularized recipient corneas which are in need of large grafts, i.e. 8.0 mm or more in diameter. The immunological privileged status of the cornea pertains only to non-vascularized recipient corneas which are transplanted with small donor buttons, because these contain very little or no HLA-DR antigenic material.

Acknowledgements

We wish to thank the staff of the Department of Immunohaematology of the Leyden University Hospital and especially Ir. Ieke Schreuder, head of the typing and screening laboratories, for the excellent technical help.

References

Braude L.S. and Chandler J.W. (1983) Corneal allograft rejection. The role of the major histocompatibility complex. Surv. of Ophthalmology 27: 290.

Ehlers N. and Ahrons S. (1971) Corneal transplantation and histocompatibility. Acta Ophthalmol. (Kbh) 49: 513.

Jones B.R. (1973) Ciba Foundation Symposium: Corneal graft failure, p. 344. Associated Scientific Publishers, Amsterdam/London/New York.

Lechler R.J. and Batchelor J.R. 1982. Restoration of immunogenicity to passenger cell-depleted kidney allografts by the addition of donor strain dendritic cells, J.Exp.Med. vol. 155: 31.

Mayer D.J., Daar A.S., Casey T.A. and Fabre J.W. (1983) Localization of HLA-A, -B, -C and -DR antigens in the human cornea. Transplantation Proceedings, XV, no. 1: 126.

Moen T., Albrechtsen D., Flatmark A., Jakobsen A., Jervell J., Halvorsen S., Solheim B. and Thorsby E. (1980) Importance of HLA-DR matching in cadaveric renal transplantation. N.Eng.J. of Medicine 303, 15: 850.

Paufique M. (1948) Les greffes de la cornée. pp. 134. Masson, Paris.

Persijn G.G., Gabb B.W., Van Leeuwen A., Nachtegaal A, Hoogeboom J., Van Rood J.J. (1978) Matching for HLA antigens of A, B and DR loci in renal transplantation by Eurotransplant. Lancet I: 1278.

Peto P., Pike M.C., Armitage P., Breslow N.E., Cox D.R., Howard S.V., Mantel N., McPherson K., Peto J. and Smith, P.G. (1976) Design and analysis of randomized clinical trials requiring prolonged observation of each patient. J.Br.J. Cancer 34: 585.

Rodriques M.M., Rowden G., Hackett J. and Bakos J.(1981) Langerhans cells in the normal conjunctiva and peripheral cornea of selected species. Invest Ophthalmol. Vis. Sci. vol. 21., 5: 759.

Van Rood J.J., Van Leeuwen A., Ploem J.S. (1976) Simultaneous detection of two cell population by two-colour fluorescence and application to recognition of B-cell determinants. Nature 262. 5571: 795.

Ting A. and Morris P.J. (1980) Powerful effect of HLA-DR matching on survival of cadaveric renal allografts. Lancet I: 282.

Völker-Dieben H.J., Kok-van Alphen C.C., Lansbergen Q. and Persijn G.G. (1982) The effect of prospective HLA-A and -B matching on corneal graft survival. Acta Ophthalmol. 60: 203.

Völker-Dieben H.J., Kok-van Alphen C.C., D'Amaro J. and de Lange P. (1984) The effect of prospective HLA-A and -B matching in 288 penetrating keratoplasties for herpes simplex keratitis. Acta Ophthalmol. in press.

CHAPTER 8

Keratoplasty in children*

Summary

Thirty-three corneal grafts in 29 children ranging in age from three to fifteen years revealed no significant difference in graft survival when compared to adult patients. Final visual acuity was mainly influenced by the amount of amblyopia. A remarkably low degree of astigmatism was observed. Pneumococcal infection and irreversible rejections were the most important complications in the postoperative period. Rejections were not observed in the 10 HLA-A and -B matched grafts. Corneal donor age did not influence corneal graft survival in children.

Introduction

Keratoplasty as a therapy for corneal opacification is generally regarded as a safe and effective procedure for the restoration of the visual acuity in adult patients. Reports on keratoplasties in children are conflicting and their results are variable. An increasing benefit has been suggested with increasing age of the patient, but, in most cases, the results remain below those obtained in adults. Children who undergo keratoplasty not only present special problems during surgery but also in the postoperative period and during the prolonged period of medical treatment.The purpose of this study is to analyze our experience in children and to report on the paediatric complications of corneal grafting.

Patients and methods

In the period from January 1976 to January 1983, 33 penetrating keratoplasties (PKP) were performed in 29 children. Their ages ranged from 3.2 years to 15 years (average 9.1 years). Of the 33 PKPs, 27 were performed in 24 children whose corneal opacities were present before the age of 6 and 6 PKP in 5 children who acquired their corneal disease after that age. Ten keratoplasties were performed with prospectively HLA-A and -B typed donors who were matched as well as possible with their recipients. HLA

* *For colour plates, see pp. 72ff.*

typings and donor selection were as described in chapter 6. All grafts were performed by only one of two surgeons (Völker-Dieben and Kok-van Alphen). Their surgical techniques were identical and conform to the method described by Harms and Mackensen (1966). Postoperative care was not changed during the period of this study and has been described (chapter 5).

Elbow restraints were not used except for one case, a keratoconus patient with Down's syndrome. Postoperative examination under general anaesthesia was only necessary in three cases. Suture removal was performed under general anaesthesia for cases up to the age of 9 years. For the older children, local anaesthesia and a careful explanation of what was going to happen was sufficient.

Twenty five patients and all graft donors were of Dutch Caucasoid origin. The four foreign patients originated from Korea, Saoudi Arabia, Suriname and Turkey.

All survival times were calculated using the actuarial life table method. The significance of the differences between the various classes were tested with X^2 statistics derived from the logrank test (Peto et al. 1976). The numbers to the right of the follow-up curves (fig. 1-4, fig. 6) indicate the number of patients at risk at the start of the study.

Results

The 33 PKPs in children from three to fifteen years consisted of 27 first grafts, 5 second grafts and one third graft. The diagnoses at the time of transplantation are listed in table 1. The two irreversibly rejected grafts were initially grafted because of herpes keratitis before 1976. Four patients were transplanted because of the failure of a previous graft. One was due to a bacterial infection in the graft. The remaining three cases were referred to us

Table 1. Diagnosis at the time of transplantation*

Diagnosis	Nr. of eyes
Herpes keratitis	11
Keratoconus	5
Burns	4
Corneal dystrophy	4
Traumatic scar	1
Bacterial keratitis	1
Dermoid cyst.	1
Irreversible rejection	2
Graft failure	4
Total	33

* for details see text

because of opaque grafts of unknown etiology. Apart from a higher number of burns in the paediatric group, no significant differences were observed when the diagnoses at the time of transplantation were compared to those in adult patients.

Corneal graft survival of the 33 PKP in children was not significantly different when compared to the graft survival of adult patients (fig. 1).

Difficulties encountered at the time of surgery are listed in table 2. Although general anaesthesia and a Flieringa ring was used in all cases, the

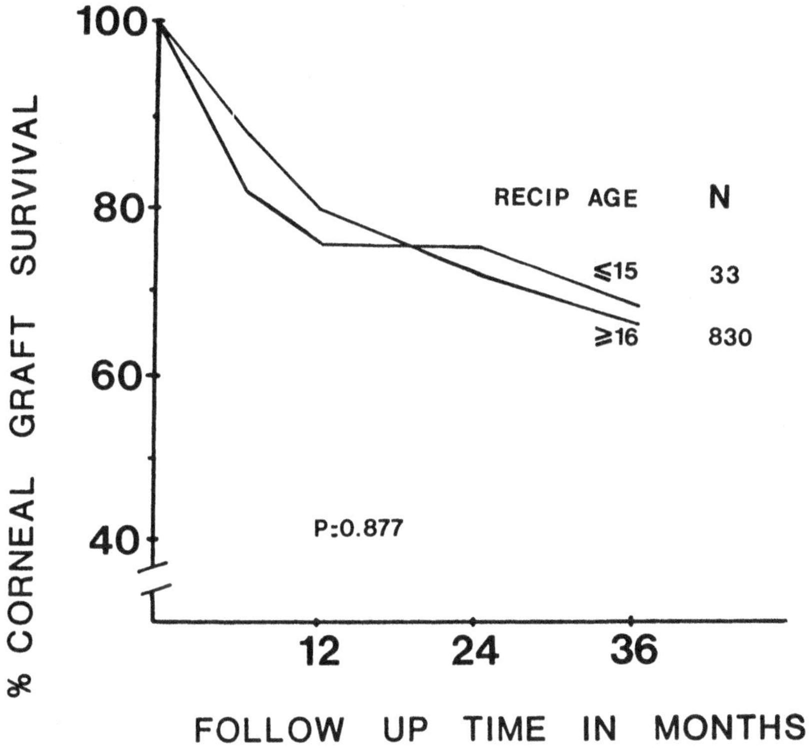

Figure 1. The influence of recipient age (≤15 = children, ≥16 = adults) on corneal graft survival.

Table 2. Difficulties encountered at the time of surgery

Anterior displacement of lens and iris	15
Fibrinous exsudates in the anterior chamber	6
Anterior synechiae	6
Cataract	2

main problem during the surgical procedure was anterior displacement of the lens and iris diaphragma. In eyes with herpetic keratitis, the fibrinous exsudation in the anterior chamber (AC) was profound. Anterior synechiae were observed in six cases and an unexpected cataract in two cases.

Complications in the postoperative period and causes of graft failure are listed in table 3. Glaucoma occurred in three cases; two of these were sufficiently treated by filtering operations, while in one case an elevated ocular pressure resulted in a clouded graft. Blunt trauma with rupture of the running suture and iris prolaps was observed in three cases. All accidents occurred in the first two months postoperatively, and in all cases the graft was resutured and the anterior chamber restored. Only one graft became opaque and a bulbar atrophy was observed later. This mentally retarded child appeared to automutilate her eye and returned with a partially loosened suture twice within the next six weeks. Suture loosening occurred in four cases in such an early post operative period that tightening of the suture was preferred above removal. Fortunately, these cases did not result in a opacification of the graft.

Corneal inflammation, either as an infiltrate or as an ulcer, was observed in seven eyes; all these infections were diagnosed within eight months postoperatively. Bacterial cultures revealed pneumococci in four cases, staphylococcus aureus in one case and pseudomonas in one case. The cornea with a pseudomonas infection was regrafted à chaud because of lysis of the first graft. The second graft is still clear after more than six years. Conservative treatment of the remaining five cases resulted in four clear grafts and one pneumococcal ulcer which healed with a macula in the graft. In one eye, a case of severe alkaline burn, a fungus infection was diagnosed and that eye developed in a bulbar atrophy. Only six immunological rejections were observed in 33 PKPs. Irreversible rejection of the graft was observed in five cases and although the patients were treated with increased amounts of dexamethason eye drops, we were not able to reverse the rejection. These five grafts became opaque. The rejection was reversed only in one case, a girl of 14 years. Systemic steroids were not used in the treatment of the rejections.

Table 3. Complication in the postoperative period and their resulting failures

	No. of complications	Resulting failures
Glaucoma	3	1
Trauma	3	1*
Suture loosening	4	–
Inflammation	7	1 + 1*
Rejection (immunological)	6	5
Cataract formation	2	–
Recurrence of herpes	1	1

* These two eyes resulted in a bulbar atrophy

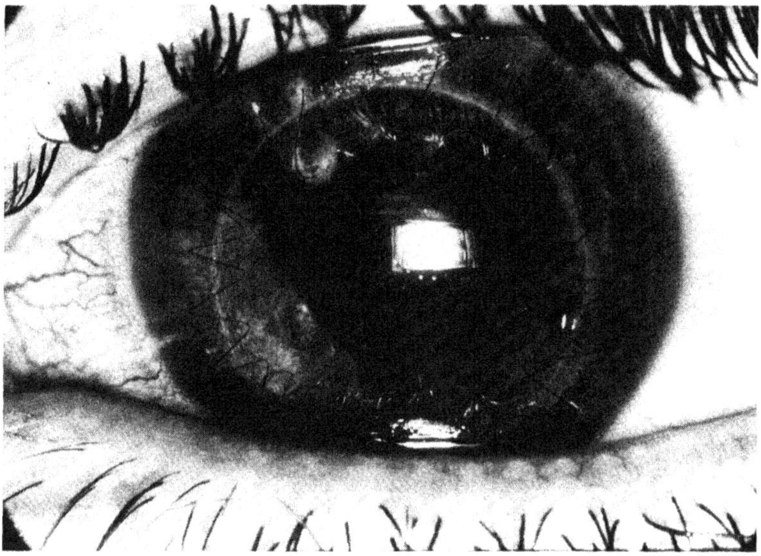

Figure 1a. Loosening of the suture of non traumatic origin.

Corneal graft rejections were not observed in the HLA-A and -B matched grafts. Table 4 summarizes the information on the 5 immunological (rejected) and the 5 non-immunologically failed grafts.

Cataract formation was seen in only two patients (see table 3). The first patient was grafted for the third time and the large amount of dexamethason eye drops may have been responsable for this cataract. Six years after the third keratoplasty had been performed, the cataract was removed extracapsulary. The graft remained transparant. The second patient with post transplantation cataract was the only one with the pseudomonas infection in the first graft and she had to be regrafted à chaud (See colour plate 3, a and b). The severe inflammation of the anterior segment in combination with large amounts of dexamethason may have caused the cataract. Cataract removal has not yet been performed since her visual acuity is still acceptable. Only one recurrence of herpes was observed. Unfortunately, that graft became opaque because of scar formation due to the herpes.

Suture removal was performed as soon as loosening of the suture without traumatic origin (fig. 1a) was observed or when increasing vascularisation of the recipient cornea became apparent. In severely vascularized eyes, because of recurrent herpes infections, we have observed small white spots where the sutures penetrate the recipient and/or the donor cornea (See colour plate 3, c and d). Whenever these microabcesses were observed, the suture was promptly removed. Suture removal was performed on an average of 6.8 months after grafting, but if indicated, as mentioned above, it was performed as soon as possible after the first 3 postoperative weeks. The necessity of suture removal on an average of 12 months in the paediatric keratoconus patients is similar to that which is commonly seen in adult patients.

Donor material selection was based on the quantity of endothelial cells. The minimal acceptable donor age was two years since below that age, there is insufficient corneal rigidity. Donor age, for the 33 paediatric keratoplaties, varied from 9 to 80 years (average 40.6 years). Corneal graft survival was not influenced by donor age in the total patient material.There was no significant difference between the survival of grafts from donors 15 years and younger as compared to those from donors older than 15 years (fig. 2). There were also no significant differences in the graft survival of grafts from young donors in young or old recipients (fig. 3) nor in the graft survival of grafts from donors older than 15 years of age in young (⩽15 years) as compared older (⩾16 years) recipients (fig. 4).

Final visual acuity was mainly influenced by the amount of amblyopia and the degree of astigmatism. Although prolonged amblyopic treatment was undertaken when necessary, full vision was never reached in these eyes. Fig. 5 summarizes the visual acuity after corneal transplantation of 22 children with a clear graft, correlated with the age of the patients at the time of transplantation. The time interval between the start of the corneal opacification and operation is indicated with a dotted line. We could not obtain reliable information about the visual acuity of one child since this keratoconus patient had Down's syndrome as well. However, his visual acuity was good enough for the child to recognize his parents from a long distance and to play with small objects. The degree of astigmatism after suture removal is of major importance for the success of amblyopia treatment. The objective corneal astigmatism measured with the keratometer ranged from zero to four diopters, with an average of 2.15 diopters in the 22 children with clear grafts. This is remarkably lower than in a random group of 25 adult patients, whose astigmatism ranged from one to 9 diopters with an average of 4.34 diopters.

Table 4. Clinical data of 5 patients with immunological graft failures and 5 patients with non-immunological failures

Patient age	sex	Cause of graft failure	graft No.	Size of graft	HLA matched	Diagnosis at transpl.	Initial diagnosis
6	♀	Rejection	1	8.0	No	Herpes	Herpes
11	♀	Rejection	1	7.0	No	Herpes	Herpes
15	♂	Rejection	1	8.5	No	Burn	Burn
14	♂	Rejection	1	7.0	No	Burn	Burn
10	♂	Rejection	1	7.5	No	Trauma	Trauma
8	♀	Glaucoma	1	7.0	Yes	Herpes	Herpes
8	♀	Trauma	2	8.0	No	Failure	Dystrophy
6	♀	Bact. infect.	1	7.0	No	Herpes	Herpes
14	♂	Fungus inf.	2	7.0	Yes	Failure	Burn
15	♀	Herpes	1	7.0	No	Herpes	Herpes

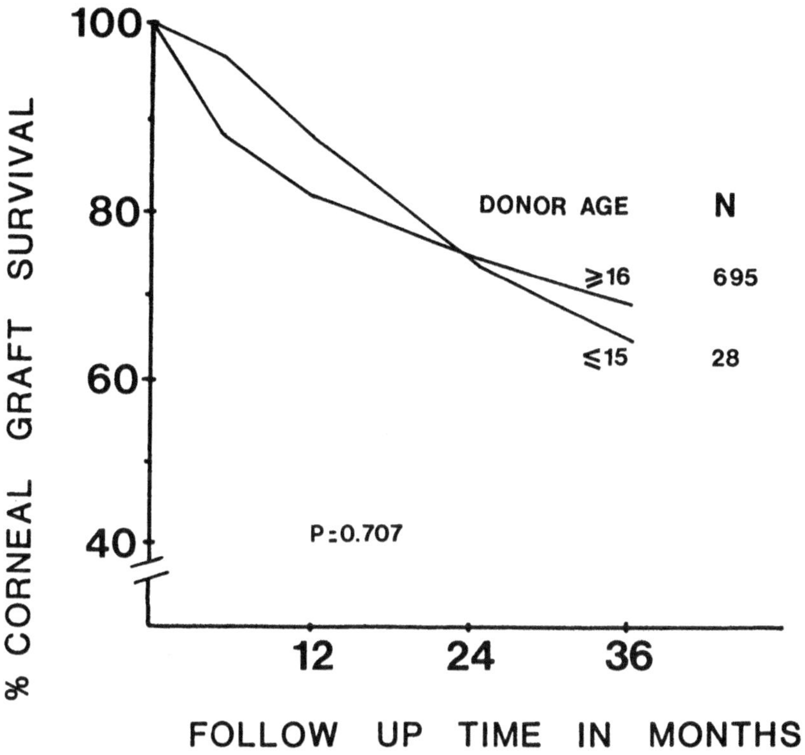

Figure 2. The influence of donor age on corneal graft survival.

Discussion

The traditional reluctance in Holland to perform keratoplasties in infants may have been responsible for the absence of very young children in this patient group. From the three children (4 x PKP) with congenital bilateral corneal dystrophy, two came from abroad, Korea and Turkey and the third child was mentally retarded. This may explain why they were not referred earlier. The child with a unilateral dermoid cyst was able to use a small paracentral part of her cornea outside the opacity after pupil dilatation. Therefore we have patched her normal eye and waited until the age of three years before performing the keratoplasty.

Our results that graft survival is not different between children and adult patients may be due to the lack of very young children. Waring and Laibson (1977) summarized their own results in paediatric keratoplasty and the results of 7 other authors. They obtained only one clear graft out of 11. In general, the results of the others are also poor and far below the results obtained in adult patients. Alberth (1980) reported that one out of 16 grafts

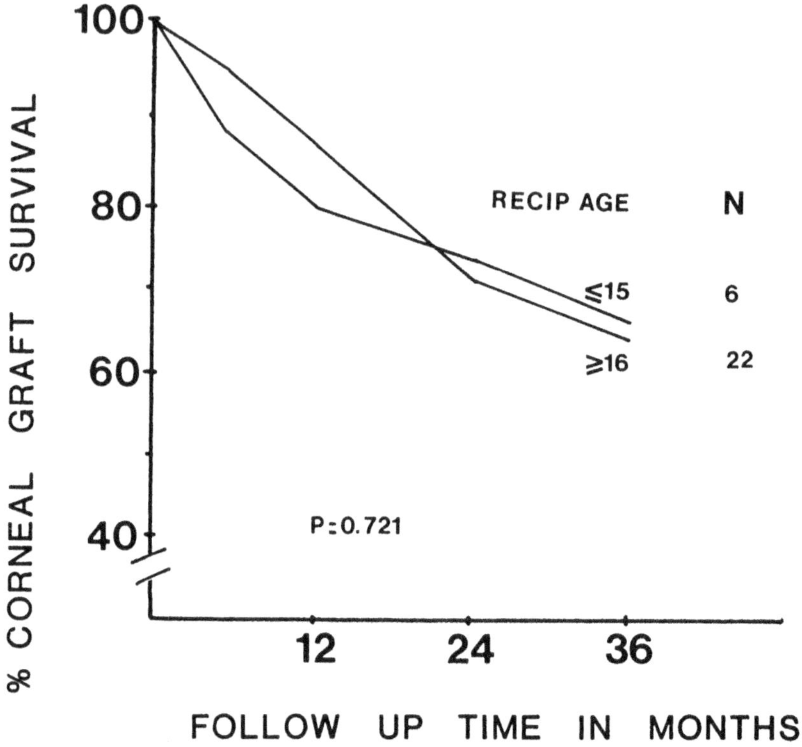

Figure 3. The influence of young donor age on corneal graft survival in children (≤15) and in adults (≥16).

remained clear. Schwanzlin et al. (1980) reported better results, 9 clear grafts out of 16 and so did Brown and Salomon (1983) who reported that 16 of 28 grafts remained clear. The ages of the children in these reports varied from two months to five years, and all patients had congenital opaque corneas. The follow-up period ranged from 6 months to 26 years. It is clear that corneal graft survival in these very young children is not comparable to our patient group.

In Beauchamp's report (1979) on 78 paediatric keratoplasties, subdivisions were made into 5 year age groups: 0-4, 5-9 etc. up to 29 years. The age groups 5-9 and 10-14 containing 20 and 11 eyes respectively can be compared to the age distribution of our patients. Unfortunately, Beauchamp reported the graft clarity in percentages of clear grafts: 55% for the age 5-9 years old children and 81% for the 10-14 years old children. The follow-up time in his study ranged from 3 months to 26 years with a mean of 4.2. years. A comparison of our results with those of Beauchamp is not possible since he did not use the actuarial life table method for calculating survival times (Peto et al. 1976). This method is the only valid method for such data since patients

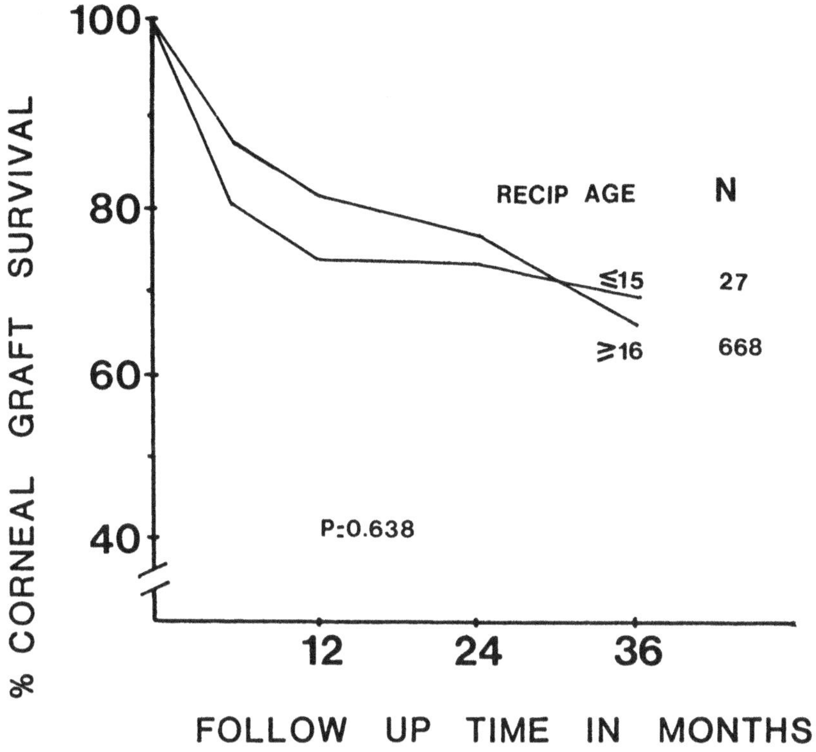

Figure 4. The influence of adult donor age on corneal graft survival in children (≤15) and in adults (≥16).

are entering the study at different periods and are followed-up for different lengths of time (Peto et al. 1976).

Anterior displacement of the iris diaphragm and of the lens was the most important complication in our patients. This observation is in concordance with all reports on pediatric keratoplasty. We would like to stress that this complication is not limited to patients under the age of 16 but, since it is the result of low scleral rigidity, it is often observed in patients over 30 years of age, especially in keratoconus patients. The use of the Flieringa ring reduces the danger of the problem of anterior displacement but does not solve it. Rapidly performed surgery and a quickly restored anterior chamber is important to prevent the formation of anterior synechiae and diminish the risk of postoperative glaucoma. The use of viscoelastic substances in the anterior chamber during surgery may be another way of solving this problem.

The postoperative course was mainly complicated by the high number of infections. Schwanzlin et al. (1980) reported 5 infections in 26 PKPs, only one case ended in a phtisis bulbi. Beauchamp (1979) reported 4 cases of

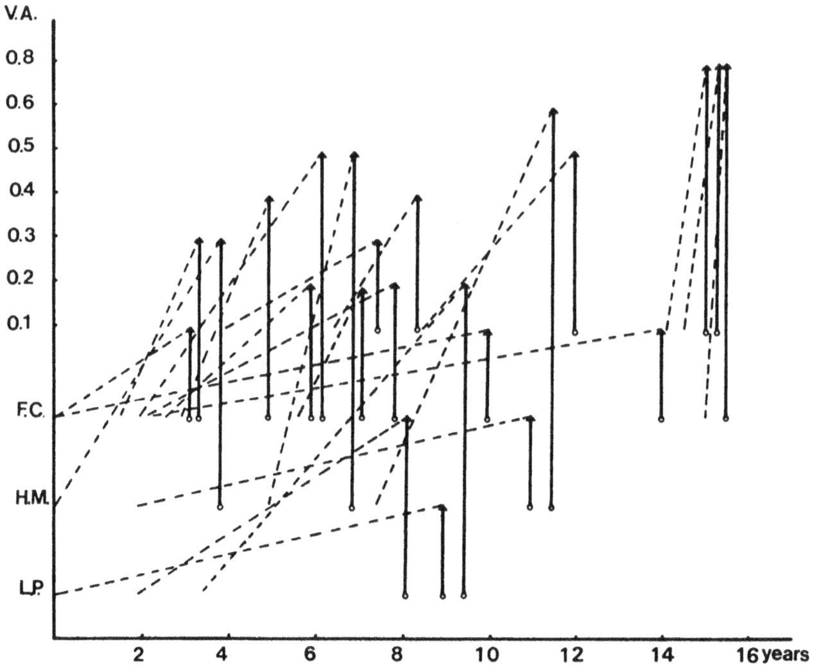

Figure 5. Visual acuity before (o.k.) and after (↑) corneal transplantation versus age at the time of operation, and time interval between start of the corneal opacification and operation (dotted line).
V.A. = visual acuity
F.C. ≙ finger counting
H.M. = hand movement
L.P. = light perception

phtisis bulbi in 42 PKPs in children up to 10 years of age. However, he did not mention how many infections were successfully treated. Our observation of 7 infections in 33 PKPs is similar to the frequency reported by Schwanzlin et al. (1980). Prompt and adequate conservative therapy cured the infections while the grafts remained clear in 5 cases. The high incidence of pneumococcal ulcers was striking. If the child suffers from upper respiratory infections, the pneumococcus is most likely to cause the corneal infiltrate. According to our experience immediate therapy with penicillin 1:100,000 E/1 ml eye drops may save the graft and the eye (See colour plate 4, a and b).

We agree with the statement of Waring and Laibson (1977) that 'the social and psychologic condition of the family often makes the difference between success and failure'. The patients' parents must be convinced of the necessity for returning to the hospital at the first sign of discomfort of the patients' eye. Tearing, photophobia or simply a 'closed eye' should warn the parents to make an early appointment.

Graft rejection was the second major complication in the postoperative period (See colour plate 4, c and d). Five of the 33 grafts became opaque for this reason, only one of them was successfully treated. We agree with Beauchamp (1979) that corneal graft rejection in children tends to be rapid and irreversible. He did not observe any reversible rejections in his patients. However, Waring and Laibson (1979) reported one successfully treated rejection in a 4 months old child and 9 irreversible rejections in 11 patients. Beauchamp (1979) reported that the usefulness of tissue typing and matching has not been established. Ehlers and Kissmeyer-Nielsen (1973), Batchelor et al. (1976) and Vannas et al. (1976) however, reported on the beneficial influence of HLA-A and -B matchting in corneal grafts although this was not statistically significant. We have observed a significantly better graft survival in HLA-A and -B matched grafts not only for vascularized corneas regardless of the initial diagnosis but also for herpes keratitis (chapter 6 and 10). Corneal graft survival in 10 matched and 23 not matched grafts demonstrated a better, but not significant, graft survival for the matched grafts (fig. 6). However, the occurrence of 5 irreversible and 1 reversible rejection in the group

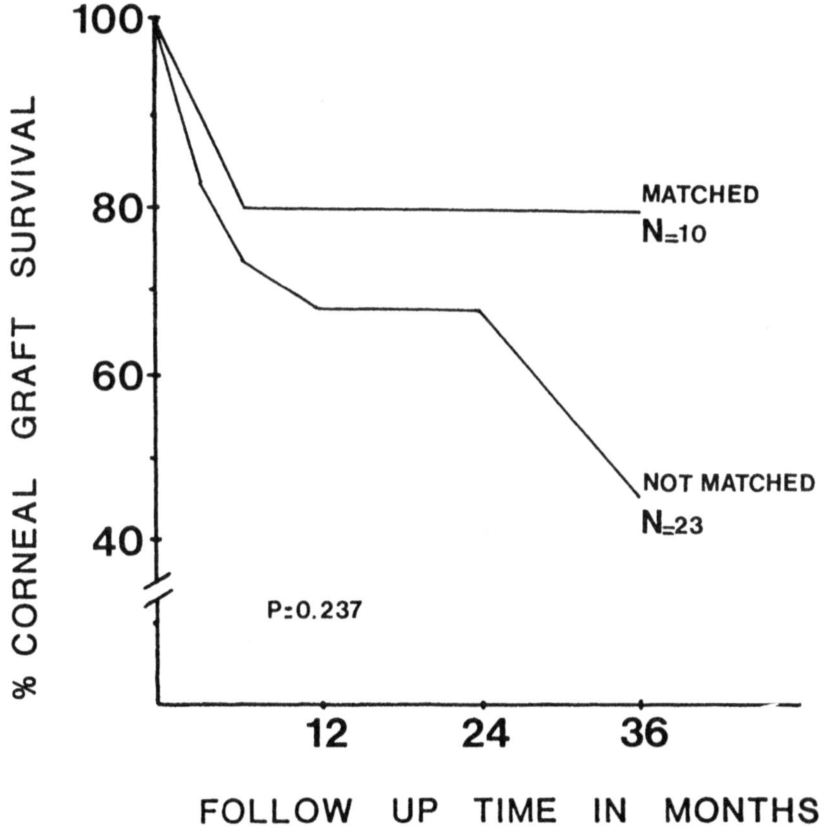

Figure 6. The effect of HLA-A and -B matching on corneal graft survival in children.

of 23 unmatched grafts versus no immunological rejection in the 10 matched grafts is noteworthy. Especially in children, who demonstrate rapid and mainly irreversible rejections, tissue typing and matching might be of value.

Wound healing appeared to be much faster in children as compared to adult patients. Rapid suture removal is indicated, especially when micro-abcesses in the cornea are observed. We confirm the statement of Brown et al. (1973) that appearance of these micro-abcesses is a clear indication for suture removal. We do not fully agree with the second indication of Brown et al. (1973) for suture removal, namely, loosening of the suture. We have made the restriction that only in the absence of trauma loosening is an indication for their removal.

The optimum donor tissue is mainly dependent on the quantity of vital endothelial cells and not dependent on the age of the donor. Specular microscopy reveals the numbers of endothelial cells, but provides us with no information about the vitality of the cells. That information can be obtained by organ culture methods which are currently being evaluated. However, our donor selection method which is based on the quantity of the endothelial cells appears to be sufficient since we have not seen any immediate graft failures in these 33 grafts. Our observation of the absence of any significant difference in graft survival in young recipients versus adult recipients when young or adult donor material was used confirms the experience of Lemp and Ralph (1975) and Beauchamp (1979).

The influence of amblyopia on the final visual acuity is well established in all reports on pediatric keratoplasty. From fig. 5 it is evident that, especially when corneal opacities occur before the age of six years, attempts should be made to shorten the duration of an opaque cornea as much as possible. In fact, tissue typing and matching may increase the waiting period since in most cases there is a longer waiting time before well matched corneas are found as compared to random corneas. Large numbers of patients may be necessary to determine if the benefits of HLA-A, -B matching overrule the disadvantage of longer waiting periods. Exchange programs for donor corneas like the one organized by the Eurotransplant Foundation, are of special importance for these paediatric patients.

The remarkably low degree of astigmatism observed in this group of pediatric patients was an unexpected observation. To our knowledge, this phenomena has never been described. A possible explanation might be the higher corneal rigidity of the adult donor corneal button as compared to the lower rigidity of the recipient ring. The recipient cornea will be molded by the shape of the donor button which is healthy corneal material with a normal curvature. That situation may justify the use of adult donor corneas instead of young donor corneas for paediatric keratoplasties.The importance of psychosocial aspects in the success rate of paediatric keratoplasties which is stressed by Waring and Laibson (1977) and by Beauchamp (1979) is certainly confirmed by us. However, the impact of a cosmetically very disturbing eye

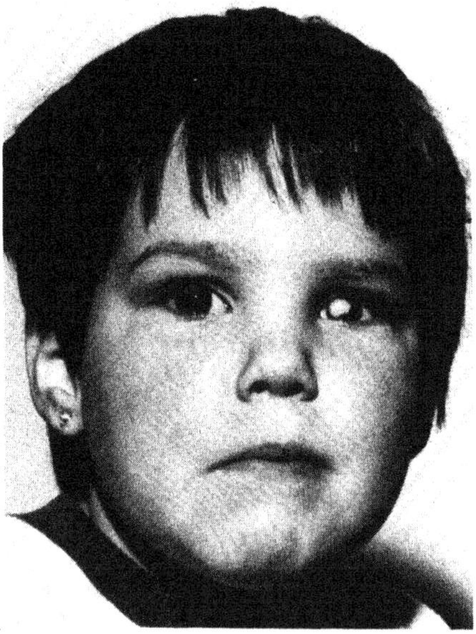

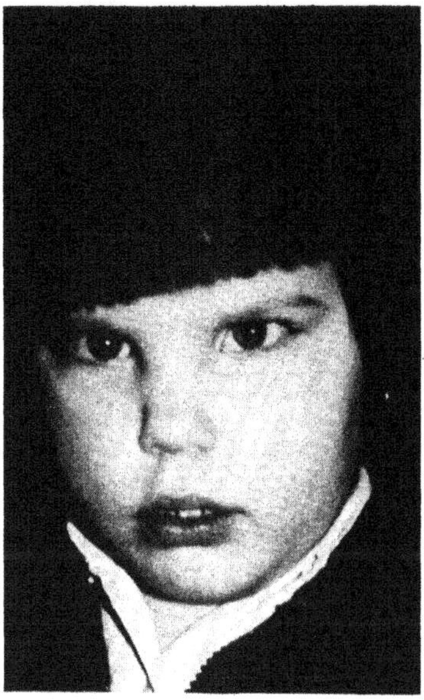

Figure 7 and 8. A cosmetically normal but functionally impaired eye (fig. 7) is preferable to a vascularised opaque cornea (fig. 8).

on the development of the child has never been mentioned. Although we are at least as conservative in the indication for keratoplasty as Alberth (1980), we feel that even a known and untreatable amblyopia should not constitute in a contra-indication for keratoplasty. A cosmetically normal but functionally impaired eye is preferable to a vascularized opaque cornea. Even a rejected cornea might be preferred above the constant recurrences of a herpes keratitis (See fig. 7 and 8).

Conclusions

- Comparable corneal graft survival in children of 3-15 years versus adult patients was observed.
- Anterior displacement of iris diaphragma and lens was the most important complication during keratoplasty in children.
- The high number of infections (7 in 33 penetrating keratoplasties) in the postoperative course are mainly due to pneumococci.
  Conservative therapy with 1:100,000 E/1 ml penicillin eye drops was the treatment of choice.
- No rejections were observed in the HLA-A and -B matched grafts, 15 irreversible and one reversible rejection were observed in the not matched group.

- No difference was observed in the survival of corneas from young (≤15 years) versus adult (≥16 years) donor nor in the survival of those 2 classes of donors corneas in young recipients versus adult recipients.
- An unexpected low degree of astigmatism was observed in this group of children.

REFERENCES

Alberth B. (1980) Keratoplastik im Säuglings- und Kindesalter. Klin. Mbl. Augenheilk. 177: 802.

Batchelor J.R., Casey T.A., Gibbs D.C., Lloyd D.F., Werb A., Prasad S.S. and James A. (1976) HLA-A matching and corneal grafting. Lancet I: 551–554.

Beauchamp G.R. (1979) Pediatric keratoplasty: problems and management. J. Ped. Ophthalmol. 16: 388.

Brown S.I., Salomon S.M. (1983) Wound healing of grafts in congenitally opaque infant corneas. Am. J. Ophthalmol. 95: 641.

Ehlers N. and Kissmeyer-Nielsen F. (1973) Influence of histo compatibility on the fate of the corneal transplant. In: Corneal graft failure, Ciba Foundation Symposium K: 307. Associated scientific Publishers, Amsterdam/London/New York.

Harms H., Mackensen H. (1966) Augenoperationen unter dem Mikroscop. p. 291. Thieme Verlag, Stuttgart.

Lemp M.A., Ralph R. (1975) Remarks on pediatric keratoplasty. II World Congress on the Cornea. Washington DC, may 1975.

Peto R., Pike M.C., Armitage P., Breslow N.E., Cox, D.R., Howard, S.V., Mantel, N., McPherson, K., Peto, J., Smith, P.G. (1976) Design and analysis of randomized clinical trials requiring prolonged observation of each patient. Br.J. Cancer 34: 585.

Schwanzlin D.J., Goldberg D.B., Brown S.I. 1980. Transplantation of congenitally opaque corneas. Ophthalmol. 87: 1253.

Vannas S., Karjalainen P., Ruusuvaara A. and Tiilikainen, A. (1976) HLA compatible donor for prevention of allograft reaction. Albrecht von Grafes Arch. Klin. Ophthalmol. 198: 217.

Waring G.O. and Laibson P.R. (1977) Keratoplasty in infants and children. Trans. Am. Acad. Ophthalmol. Otolaryngol. 83: 283. March-April.

CHAPTER 9

The influence of intraocular lenses on corneal graft survival in patients with endothelial decompensation*

Summary

Reexamination of the fate of 136 corneal grafts in bullous keratopathy (secondary endothelial decompensation) revealed a decreased, but not significant, graft survival of those grafts compared to the total of 572 grafts in patients with other diagnoses. There was also a decreased but not significant graft survival when compared to the survival of the grafts for Fuchs' dystrophy (primary endothelial decompensation).

A statistically significant decreased graft survival (p=0.015) was observed when corneal grafts performed in pseudophakic eyes with secondary endothelial decompensation were compared to those performed in aphakic eyes with secondary endothelial decompensation. An immunological explanation for this difference was not detected. The influence of an intraocular lens on corneal graft survival was analyzed. Indications for removing or retaining the intraocular lens at the time of graft surgery are reported.

Introduction

Corneal endothelial decompensation, resulting in the occurrence of bullous keratopathy, is always due to a decrease in the number of normally functioning endothelial cells to less than the critical number of cells required to maintain the corneal clarity (Maurice, 1968). Endothelial cell damage at the time of cataract surgery, whether or not followed by an intraocular lens implantation, has been reported by several authors (see review by Leonard and Rommel, 1982). Factors other than endothelial cell loss at the time of surgery may influence endothelial decompensation, such as intraocular lens subluxation with permanent or intermittent endothelial touch, peripheral anterior synechiae, extrusion of the vitreous into the anterior chamber, secondary glaucoma and chronic iritis.

In many cases of bullous keratopathy, the intraocular lens may be responsable for the endothelial decompensation (Bourne and Kaufman, 1976). We reviewed our series of corneal grafts in patients with pseudophakic and aphakic bullous keratopathy in order to see whether or not their survival was influenced by an intraocular lens. The aim of the study was to determine indications for removing or retaining the intraocular lens at the time of graft surgery.

* *For colour plates, see pp. 72ff.*

Material and methods

Between January 1976 and January 1982, 708 full thickness keratoplasties were performed. The initial indications for grafting are listed in table 1. Of the 708 grafts, 136 were performed because of bullous keratopathy or secondary endothelial decompensation (S.E.D.). The term S.E.D. is preferred above bullous keratopathy in order to distinguish secondary endothelial decompensation following intraocular surgery from the primary endothelial decompensation (P.E.D.) or Fuchs' dystrophy. These corneas are decompensated without surgical intervention.

The follow-up period ranges from 6 months to 6 years, average 30.4 months. The 129 patients (136 eyes with S.E.D.) were referred by 43 different ophthalmic surgeons. All corneal transplants were performed only by 2 surgeons (Völker-Dieben and Kok-van Alphen). Our surgical techniques were identical. Technique, postoperative treatment and donor selection were as described earlier (chapter 5). A larger trephine (0.5 mm) was used routinely to cut the donor tissue than was used to cut the recipient opening in all pseudophakic and aphakic eyes. Anterior vitrectomy was performed with the manual technique. Cellulose sponges were touched to the free vitreous strands in the anterior chamber and retracted slightly above the plane of the iris, scissors were used to cut the vitreous in the pupil. All free vitreous in the anterior chamber was removed. The ages of the patients ranged from 26 to 87 years with an average of 71.4 years. Sex distribution in the patients with endothelial decompensation was 74 females and 55 males. All patients and graft donors were of the Dutch Caucasoid origin. All graft survival times were calculated using the actuarial life table method as described earlier (chapter 5). The numbers to the right of the follow-up curves (fig. 1 - 3) indicate the numbers of patients at risk at the start of the study.

S.E.D. was observed in 85 pseudophakic eyes, 44 aphakic eyes, 4 injured (aphakic) eyes and 3 phakic glaucoma eyes, in which glaucoma surgery had been performed. Nine of the 44 aphakic eyes had been pseudophakic previously, the intraocular lens (I.O.L.) was removed by the referring

Table 1. The initial indication for grafting

Diagnosis	Number of cases
Herpes keratitis	238
Secondary Endothelial Decompensation (S.E.D.)	136
Primary Endothelial Decompensation (P.E.D.)	45
Keratoconus	91
Other dystrophies	41
Injuries	22
Burns	22
Other	113
Total	708

ophthalmologist in an attempt to arrest progression of the corneal oedema. All lenses used in the initital surgery were of the iris fixation or iridocapsular type. Thirteen cataract extractions were performed with the extracapsular method and 72 with the intracapsular extraction method.

The 85 pseudophakic eyes contained the following lens types: 41 Binkhorst lenses (7 two loop and 34 four loop lenses) and 42 Worst medaillon lenses (22 sutured on the iris with 10x0 nylon, 5 lenses iris fixed with stainless steel and 15 lenses with a platina safety pin), one kite type lens and one lobster claw lens. Seven I.O.L. were removed at the time of graft surgery, thereby reducing the initial number of 85 pseudophakic eyes to 78 and increasing the number of aphakic eyes post-operatively to 55 (See colour plate 5, a and b).

The average interval between cataract extraction and the development of S.E.D. was 1.3 years. The average interval between the date of cataract extraction and perforating keratoplasty was 3.4 years. Therefore the average duration of the S.E.D. was 2.1 years. Whether the initial surgical procedure was an intracapsular or an extracapsular cataract extraction resulted in only a slight difference in interval between cataract extraction and S.E.D.: 18.4 months for the 72 intracapsular extractions and 11.1 months for the 13 extracapsular cataract extractions.

Results

The 2 year survival of 136 corneal grafts in eyes with S.E.D. was found to be lower (59.7%) compared to the total of 572 grafts performed because of other indications, 76.1% at 2 years (fig. 1).

In corneas with S.E.D., the entire endothelial cell layer is decompensated. In the grafting procedure only the central part of the cornea is removed. Migration of endothelial cells from the grafted corneal button towards the remaining decompensated periferal corneal rim could be the cause of a graft failure. If so, no difference in graft survival rate in eyes with S.E.D. and P.E.D. should be expected. Comparison of the graft survival rate of the 136 eyes with S.E.D. and the 45 eyes with P.E.D. demonstrated a lower graft survival at 2 years, 59.7% for the S.E.D. compared to 73.7% for the P.E.D. (fig. 2).

There is no agreement on the influence of I.O.L. on corneal graft survival. The 2 year graft survival rate in the 78 pseudophakic eyes (P.S.P.H.) was 48.5% compared to the 72.5% survival in the 55 aphakic eyes (A.P.H.) (fig. 3). The causes of this significant difference ($p = 0.015$) in graft survival are listed in Table 2. Raised intraocular pressure (I.O.P.) was found in 17 pseudophakic and 12 aphakic eyes after keratoplasty. In 4 pseudophakic and 3 aphakic eyes we were unable to control the intraocular eye pressure with conservative antiglaucoma therapy. Cyclocryo therapy was performed in 4 cases, while filtering glaucoma surgery was performed in 2 cases. One patient

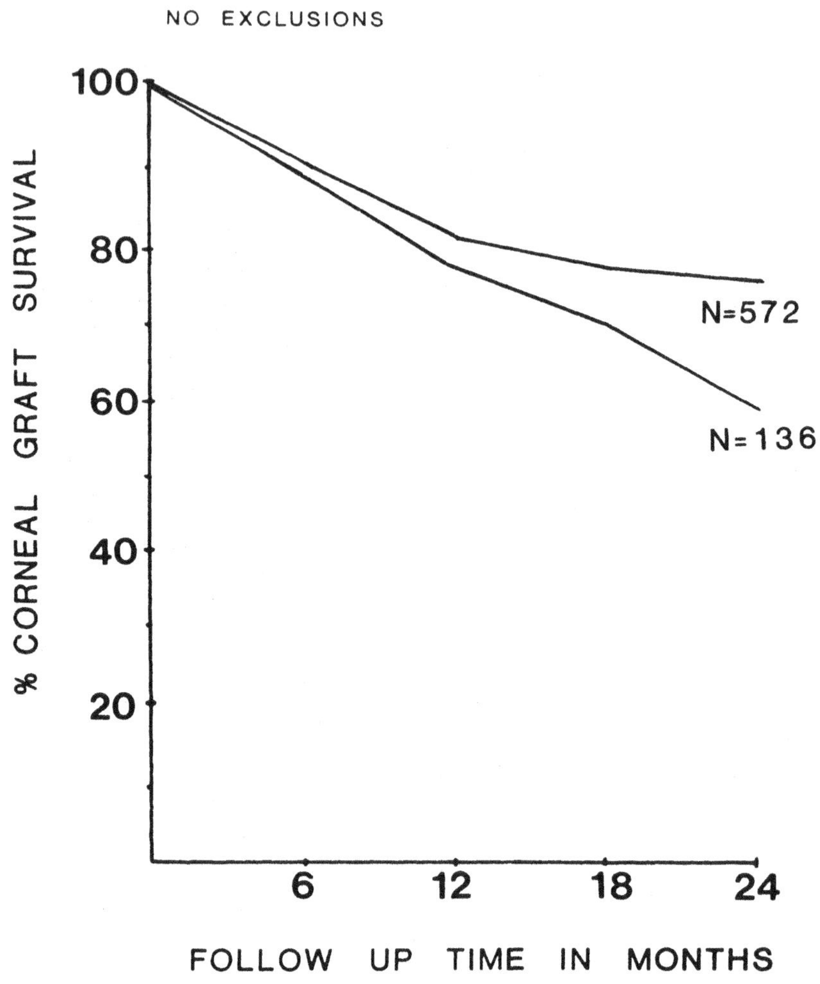

Figure 1. The influence of the initial diagnosis Secondary Endothelial Decompensation (N=136) versus 'non' Secondary Endothelial Decompensation (N=572).

refused surgical glaucoma therapy because her aphakic eye already had a very poor visual acuity and she had no complaints from the raised intraocular pressure. Six grafts became clouded by glaucoma (3 aphakic and 3 pseudophakic eyes). In eight cases the cause of graft failure was touch of the I.O.L. to the endothelial cell layer of the cornea, either the transplanted corneal button or the recipient corneal rim. Slowly progressive late corneal oedema (12 months p.o.) was observed in 7 pseudophakic eyes and 1 aphakic eye. No signs of permanent or intermittent touch of the I.O.L. could be detected in these 7 pseudophakic eyes. In none of those cases were signs of

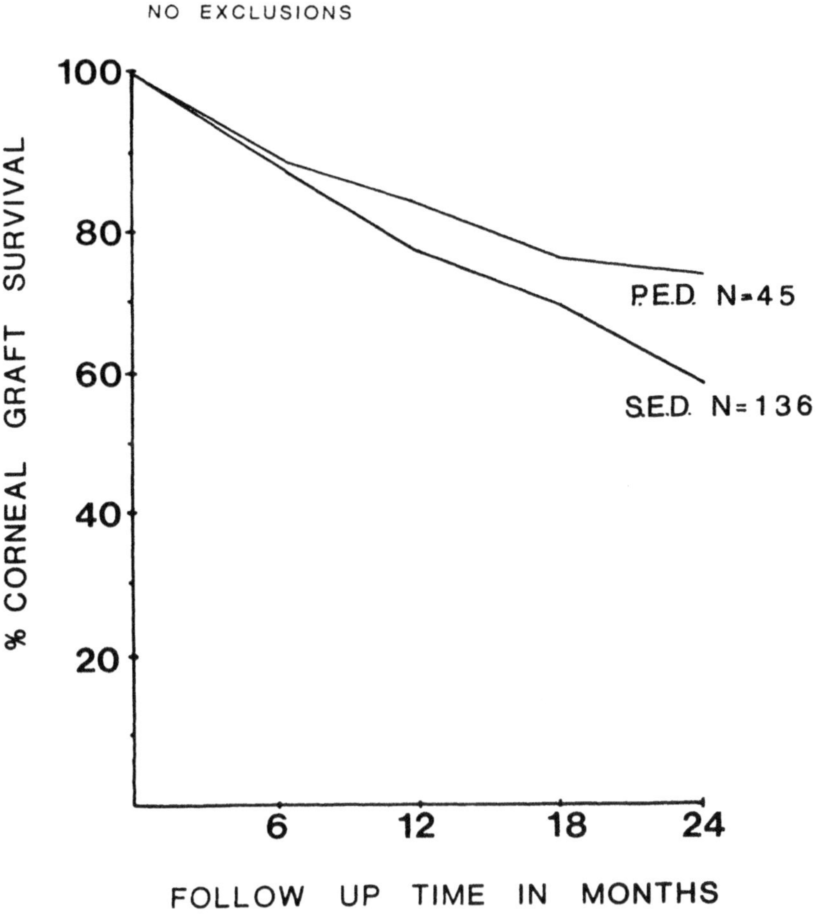

Figure 2. The influence of the initial diagnosis Secondary Endothelial Decompensation versus Primary Endothelial Decompensation.

immunological rejection observed. Graft failure caused by irreversible rejection was less than 10% after 2 years. Four rejected corneas were found in the pseudophakic eyes and 6 in the aphakic eyes.

The problems encountered at the time of transplantation have to be considered as well when analyzing the causes of graft failure (Table 3). It is highly probable that patients develop corneal decompensation because of complicated cataract surgery with or without intraocular lens implantation. In the larger part of the cases, more than one problem was encountered in one eye at the time of transplantation. Thirty-nine I.O.L. were decentered, and 21 of them were attached to the cornea. A tilted I.O.L. was observed in 3 eyes.

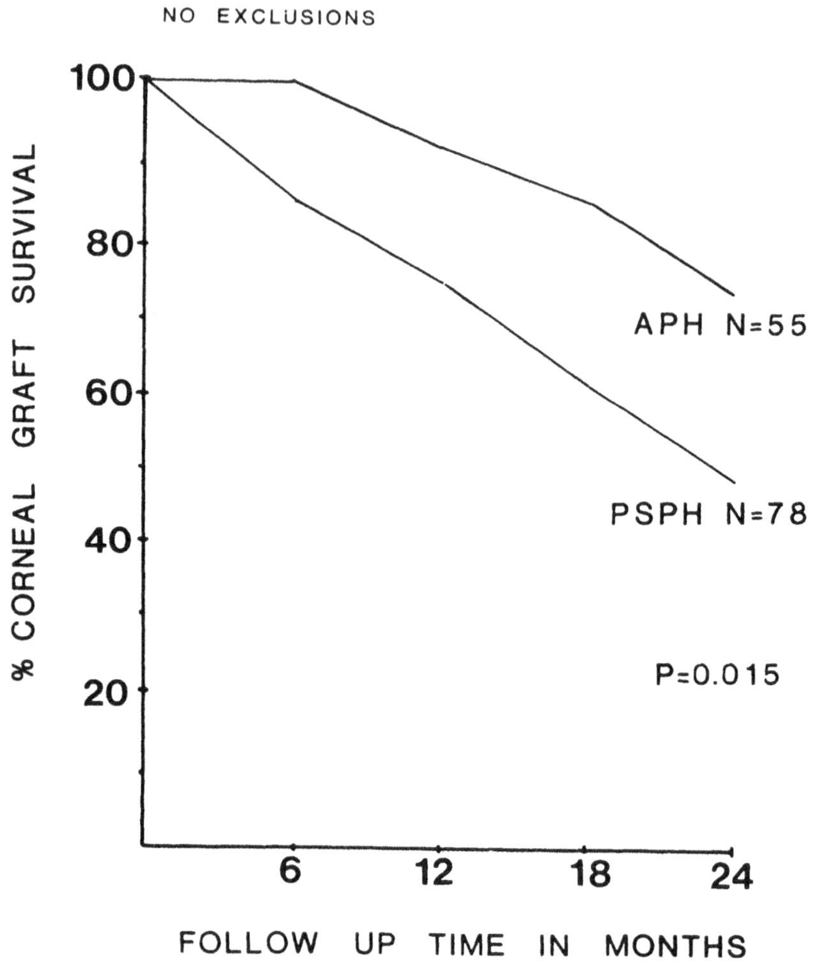

Figure 3. The influence of pseudophakia or aphakia and Secondary Endothelial Decompensation

Table 2. Causes of graft failure in 133 S.E.D. grafts

	Pseudophakic	Aphakic
I.O.P. raised	3	3
I.O.L. touch	8	
Late corneal edema	7	1
Rejection	4	6
Infection	1	
Trauma	1	
Retinal surgery		1

Table 3. Problems encountered at the time of transplantation in 136 S.E.D. grafts

	Pseudophakic	Aphakic
I.O.L. attached to the cornea	21	
Decentered I.O.L.	39	
Tilted I.O.L.	3	
Vitreous in A.C. through iridectomy	32	24
Vitreous in A.C. through pupil	38	43
Anterior iris synechiae	19	10

Vitreous in the anterior chamber (A.C.) was observed in pseudophakic eyes as well as in aphakic eyes. The entrance to the anterior chamber was formed either by the pupil or by an (excessively large) iridectomy. Anterior iris synechiae existed in 19 pseudophakic and 10 aphakic eyes.

Cystoid macular oedema (C.M.E.), ophthalmoscopically determined, was present in 21 of the 54 pseudo phakic eyes with a clear graft. There were 40 aphakic eyes with a clear graft, 17 with C.M.E. It is interesting to note that C.M.E. was observed in 10 of the 16 aphakic eyes which had been previously pseudophakic - the I.O.L. was removed either before graft surgery (9 cases) or at the time of surgery (7 cases).

Discussion

Several recent publications reported a high percentage of clear grafts after penetrating keratoplasty performed for pseudophakic or aphakic S.E.D. (see Table 4). We were interested in determining if there was any agreement between their results and ours. However, this was not possible because of the following reasons. Firstly, there was no agreement on diagnostic classification of patients. Secondly, the method used to evaluate the percentage of clear grafts was not appropriate to the data. An actuarial life table method, as used in the evaluation of renal transplants, is the only valid method for such data, since patients are entering at different periods and are followed up for different lengths of time (Peto et al. 1976). Although Stanley et al. (1981) did not perform a life table analysis of the results of 73 consequitive transplants in aphakic eyes with S.E.D., they did follow up all of their patients for a minimum of 24 months. Their report of 78% clear grafts at 24 months is perhaps comparable to our finding of 72.5% graft survival rate at the end of the same time period.

Arentsen and Laibson (1982) reported only 1 case of postoperative I.O.L. touch to the cornea. It was not clear whether or not graft failure was caused by that complication. Of the 40 initially pseudophakic eyes, 18 I.O.L. were removed and 22 remained in the eye.

Neither Charlton et al. (1981) nor Waltman (1981) reported I.O.L. touch after penetrating keratoplasty. Charlton removed 11 of the 19 I.O.L. and

Table 4. Overview of reports on graft survival in patients with endothelial decompensation

Author	Nr. of grafts S.E.D.			Nr. of grafts P.E.D.			Nr. of grafts OTHER	Follow-up in months	% Clear grafts			
AUTHOR												
Arentsen 1982	–	22	18	–	–	–		6 or more av. 18	100?			
Charlton 1982	–	13**	11	–	8	10	51	12 to 20	85 (all patients)			
Olson 1979	–	–	23	–	–	20	–	12	95 (all patients)			
Stanley 1981	–	–	73	–	–	–	–	24	78			
Waltman 1981	–	31	5	–	–	–	–	12 or more	89.9			
Völker-Dieben	3	78	55	19	12	13	–	6 to 72	*S.E.D.*	59.7*	*P.E.D.*	73.7*
(this study)								av. 30.4	ph.	–	ph.	82.2*
									psph.	48.5*	psph.	65.5*
									aph.	72.5*	aph.	66.6*
postop. status	ph.	psph.	aph.	ph.	psph.	aph.						

* Data based on actuarial life tables

** 13 = 8 I.O.L. + 5 secondary I.O.L.

ph = phakic psph = pseudophakic aph = aphakic

S.E.D. = secondary endothelial decompensation (bullous keratopathy) P.E.D. = primary endothelial decompensation (Fuchs dystrophy) inserted 5 I.O.L. in aphakic eyes at the time of grafting. Waltman removed 5 of the 36 I.O.L. at the time of transplantation. In our study of 78 transplanted pseudophakic eyes, 8 grafts failed because of I.O.L. touch. The significant difference in graft survival rate of 48.5% for the pseudophakic eyes with S.E.D. and 72.5% for the aphakic eyes with S.E.D. emphasizes the need for careful determination of the influence of the I.O.L. on graft survival.

The I.O.L. position was evaluated at the time of transplantation and, if necessary, an anterior vitrectomy was performed, either through the iridectomy or underneath the I.O.L. Anterior synechiae from I.O.L. to cornea and/or from iris to cornea were loosened. During keratoplasty, the anterior loops of the 4 loop Binkhorst lenses were cut off in 4 cases (See colour plate 4, c and d). In 7 cases removal of the lens was the only solution. In spite of all of our efforts, 8 grafts failed because of renewed I.O.L. touch. This experience has taught us that we have been too optimistic about the techniques for good centration of a decentered I.O.L. (See colour plate 6, b, c and d).

Raised intraocular pressure after graft surgery was reported by Arentsen, Charlton, Olson and Stanley. Eighteen out of 40 eyes with S.E.D., 3 out of 24, 3 out of 23 and 12 out of 73 eyes with S.E.D. respectively. Arentsen did not differentiate between pseudophakic and aphakic eyes, the latter three authors reported raised I.O.P. only in aphakic eyes. They reported no graft failures in these cases. We observed 17 cases of raised I.O.P. in 78 pseudophakic eyes and 12 cases in 55 aphakic eyes. No significant difference between the 2 groups was observed. Finally, 3 grafts in pseudophakic and 3 grafts in aphakic eyes clouded for this reason.

The first 5 authors listed in Table 4 mention very low incidences of immunological graft failure without citing the data. No comparison with our material could be made because of the lack of comparable follow-up times. We observed 4 irreversibly rejected corneas in 78 pseudophakic eyes and 6 in the 55 aphakic ones. Although the percentage of irreversible rejected corneas is twice as high in the aphakic as in the pseudophakic eyes, the main cause of graft failure in the pseudophakic eyes is I.O.L. touch. Those grafts clouded within the first postoperative year. It is evident that it is difficult to diagnose an irreversible rejection in an already opaque graft. Therefore, we may be missing that diagnosis in pseudophakic eyes. Hence, no firm conclusions can be drawn from the different numbers of rejected grafts in the pseudophakic and aphakic eyes.

Slowly progressive late corneal oedema without signs of graft rejection was observed in 7 pseudophakic and 1 aphakic eye. The intracapsular cataract extraction method was used for these 8 cases. Pronounced pseudophakodonesis/iridonesis was noted in all of those cases. As Binkhorst (1980) explained in his theoretical considerations regarding intracapsular versus extracapsular cataract extraction, an intraocular lens may aggravate the consequences of the 'Barrier Deprivation Syndrome'. Iris-fixed lenses increase endophthalmodonesis after intracapsular cataract extraction.

Constant aqueous turbulence may cause a continuous loss of endothelial cells. The explanation for these oedematous grafts might be the 'turbulence endotheliopathy'. If the secondary endothelial decompensation and the endothelial decompensation in the corneal graft occur in a slowly progressive manner, without any touch of the I.O.L. to the endothelial cell layer, the I.O.L. should be stablelized (Worst, 1979) (See colour plate 6, a). This procedure should be performed preferably before transplantation in order to observe the effect on the pseudophakodonesis. If the pseudophakodonesis still persists, then the I.O.L. should be removed at the time of transplantation.

C.M.E. was reported by many authors to be the most common explanation for the disappointing visual acuity after penetrating keratoplasty because of S.E.D. Kok-van Alphen and Völker-Dieben (1979) reported that the most favourable results with respect to the visual acuity are obtained if the corneal graft is performed within 9 months after the onset of the S.E.D. They suggested that prolonged irritation of the anterior segment by keratitis bullosa (S.E.D.) may result in cystoid macula oedema in the retina. Charlton (1981) reported better visual acuity after grafting pseudophakic eyes as compared to grafting aphakic eyes with S.E.D.

The time interval between cataract surgery (and lens implantation) and transplantation was 2.6 years for the pseudophakic eyes and 6.8 years for the aphakic eyes. However, the percentage of C.M.E. in both groups was almost the same, 36% and 35% respectively. Waltman and Arentsen suggested that disturbing the vitreous at the time of transplantation may cause C.M.E. We observed C.M.E. in 21 (38.8%) of the 54 pseudophakic eyes with a clear graft and 17 (40%) of the 42 aphakic eyes with a clear graft. However, if the aphakic eyes are divided into those which had been pseudophakic previously or not, then it appears that in the 16 eyes from which the I.O.L. was removed, 10 cases (62.5%) of C.M.E. were found while only 7 cases (29.2%) of C.M.E. were observed in the 24 eyes which had always been aphakic. Since I.O.L. removal always requires vitrectomy, we agree with the suggestion of Waltman (1981) and Arentsen and Laibson (1982) that disturbing the vitreous may cause C.M.E. However, our results are not in concordance with the suggestion of Charlton et al. (1981) that an I.O.L can be successfully removed at the time of keratoplasty without reducing the prognosis for recovery of visual acuity. However, they confirm the result of Arentsen and Laibson (1982) who found a statistically significant improvement in visual acuity in the group with a retained I.O.L. compared to the group where the I.O.L. was removed.

Conclusions

- Secondary endothelial decompensation after cataract surgery with or without an intraocular lens (I.O.L.)implantation is irreversible.

- Removal of the intraocular lens through the cataract incision does not arrest the progress of the endothelial decompensation.
- Long standing endothelial decompensation may cause cystoid macular oedema (C.M.E.). Efforts should be made to perform perforating keratoplasty as soon as possible in order to reduce the time during which the eye remains in an irritated state.
- Vitreous manipulation at the time of transplantation may cause cystoid macular oedema.
- The final decision regarding the removal or retention of the intraocular lens in eyes with secondary endothelial decompensation should be made at the time of transplantation.
- The survival of grafts in patients with S.E.D. was lower, but not significantly different from that of grafts in non-decompensated recipients, or in P.E.D. recipients. Graft survival in S.E.D. patients was lower in those with intraocular lenses (pseudophakic) than in the aphakic eyes.

Arguments in favour of removing the intraocular lens (I.O.L.) are:

1. A better graft survival at 2 years in aphakic eyes compared to pseudophakic eyes (72.5% versus 48.5%, overall $p = 0.015$).
2. Anterior synechiae, loosened in order to center an intraocular lens tend to adhere again in the post-operative period.
3. Intermittent touch of the platinum fixation clip of the intraocular lens leads to recurrence of endothelial decompensation.
4. Pronounced pseudophakodonesis without observable intermittent touch of the intraocular lens combined with late corneal oedema of the graft ('turbulence endotheliopathy') leads to recurrent endothelial decompensation.

Arguments in favour of retaining the intraocularlens (I.O.L.) are:

1. Prevention of new surgical trauma with a certain disturbance of the vitreous which may cause cystoid macular oedema.
2. The attainment of a deep anterior chamber and well centered intraocular lens without anterior synechiae after evaluation of the lens position during transplantation.
3. In cases of intermittent touch caused by the anterior loops of the intraocular lens, loops should be severed.
4. In the event of macular disease prior to grafting, the aphakic spectacle ring scotoma adds to the problems of the patient with already a loss of central vision.

Finally, the disappointing visual acuity after keratoplasty because of secondary endothelial decompensation (S.E.D.) should not discourage surgeons from operating on these patients. In the absence of grafting, progressive endothelial decompensation will not only cause a blurred vision and light sensitiveness but also broken corneal epithelial bullae will inevitably add severe pain to their complaints.

References

Arentsen J.J. and Laibson P.R. (1982) Surgical management of pseudophakic corneal edema: complications and visual results following penetrating keratoplasty. Ophthalmic Surgery 13: 371-373.

Binkhorst C.D. (1980) Corneal and retinal complications after cataract extraction. Ophthalmology 87: 609.

Bourne W.M. and Kaufman H.E. (1976) Endothelial damage associated with intraocular lenses. Am.J.Ophthal. 81: 482-485.

Charlton K.H., Binder P.S. and Perl T. (1981) Visual prognosis in pseudophakic corneal transplant. Ophthalmic Surgery 12: 411-419.

Kok-van Alphen C.C. and Völker-Dieben H.J. (1979) Corneal dystrophy following lens implantation. Doc. Ophthalmol. 48 (2): 243-250.

Leonard P. and Rommel J. (1982) Lens implantation, 30 years of progress. Dr. W. Junk Publishers, The Hague, Boston, London.

Maurice D.M. (1968) Cellular membrane activity in the corneal endothelium of the intact eye. Experientia 24: 1094.

Olson R.J., Waltman S.R., Mattingly T.P. and Kaufman H.E. (1979) Visual results after penetrating keratoplasty for aphakic bullous keratopathy and Fuchs' dystrophy. Am.J.Ophthalm. 88: 1000-1004.

Peto R., Pike M.C., Armitage P., Breslow P., Breslow N.E, Cox P.R., Howard S.V, Mantel N., McPherson K., Peto J. and Smith P.G. (1976) Design and analysis of randomized clinical trials requiring prolonged observation of each patient. I. Br.J. Cancer 34: 585.

Stanley Muenzler W. and Harms W.K. (1981) Visual prognosis in aphakic bullous keratopathy treated by penetrating keratoplasty: a retrospective study of 73 cases. Ophthalmic Surgery 12: 210-212.

Waltman S.R. (1981) Penetrating keratoplasty for pseudophakic bullous keratopathy. Achr. Ophthalmol.99: 415-416.

Worst J. (1979) Premier festival du film sur l'implantation du linse. Cannes.

CHAPTER 10

The effect of prospective HLA-A and -B matching in 288 penetrating keratoplasties for herpes simplex keratitis*

Summary

A retrospective review of 288 penetrating keratoplasties (PKP) for herpes simplex keratitis demonstrated a 60% survival of clear grafts at three years.

A highly significant difference in corneal graft survival in moderately or severely vascularised corneas (57.1% at three years) versus non or slightly vascularised corneas (82.8% at three years) was observed (p=0.009). Prospectively HLA-A and -B matched grafts in vascularised corneas revealed a significantly improved graft survival when compared to unmatched grafts (p=0.035).

Corneal graft survival in eyes grafted 'à chaud' was not significantly below the graft survival of vascularised corneas with a clinically non-active herpetic corneal disease.

Recurrence of herpes simplex in the graft was observed in an earlier postoperative period in HLA-A and -B matched grafts as compared to unmatched grafts (p=0.0004).

Introduction

Recurrent herpes simplex virus (HSV) keratitis leads to corneal scarring and impaired visual acuity. The frequent recurrences of HSV keratitis and the ensuing necessity of continuous supervision by the ophthalmologist constitute a serious handicap on the social acitivities of patients. For many patients, a corneal transplant is the only chance for restoring vision and reestablishing their normal social lives. Unfortunately, the possibility of graft opacification, of which the main cause is immunologic rejection of the graft, remains. The aim of this study is to determine whether or not prospective HLA-A and -B matching has a beneficial effect on corneal graft survival.

Materials and methods

In the period from January 1976 to January 1983, 858 penetrating keratoplasties (PKP) were performed, 288 because of recurrent HSV keratitis. In 250 cases, the diseased corneas were moderately or severely vascularised. Twenty six corneas had to be grafted à chaud because of perforation or descemetocele. The remaining 224 grafts were performed in

* *For colour plates, see pp. 72ff.*

eyes clinically without active herpes infection at the time of surgery. The visual acuity of the eyes before grafting was always 0.1 or less. Of the 288 keratoplasties 110 were performed with prospectively HLA-A and -B typed donors who were matched as well as possible with the recipients. HLA typings and donor cornea selection were as previously described (chapter 6).

All grafts were performed only by two surgeons (Völker-Dieben and Kok-van Alphen). Their surgical techniques were identical and conformed to the method described by Harms and Mackensen (1966). Postoperative care was not changed during the period of this study and was as previously described (chapter 6).The ages of the 267 patients (288 eyes), 179 men and 88 women, ranged from 4 to 83 years (mean age 56.3 years). Only 11 patients were 15 years of age or younger. The period of herpetic recurrences before grafting ranged from 2 to 65 years (mean duration 14.5 years). All patients were treated pre-operatively with the antiviral eye drops Idoxuridinum (IDU) 1mg and trifluorthymidine (TFT) 1% and corticosteroid eye drops. Antiviral therapy was not continued postoperatively.

All patients and graft donors were of Dutch Caucasoid origin. All survival times were calculated using the actuarial life table method. The significance of the differences between the various classes were tested with X^2 statistics derived from the logrank test (Peto et al. 1976). The numbers to the right of the follow-up curves (fig. 1-3) indicate the number of patients at risk at the start of the study.

Results

Corneal graft survival in recurrent HSV keratitis was lower (75.0%, 68.2% and 60.4% at one, two and three years) than in eyes grafted for non herpetic diseases (81.9%, 73.7% and 70.9% at one, two and three years) (overall p=0.050) (fig. 1).

Of the 288 grafts, 250 were performed in moderately or severely vascularised corneas and 38 in non or slightly vascularised corneas. The graft survival in vascularised corneas was significantly lower (72.5%, 65.3% and 57.1% at one, two and three years) than in non or slightly vascularised corneas (91.1%, 87.4% and 82.8% at the same time interval) (overall p=0.009) (fig. 2).

HLA typed and matched donor corneas were used for patients with vascularised corneas. The matched corneal grafts had a significantly better survival as compared to the unmatched grafts in vascularised corneas: 80.5%, 74.1% and 67.2% at one, two and three years for the matched grafts, versus 66.7%, 59.0% and 50.3% for the unmatched group in the same time intervals, p=0.035 (fig. 3).

In 26 cases, it was imperative to perform the corneal graft à chaud. All of those corneas were either perforated or with a descemetocele (See colour plate 7, a, b, c and d). They were all severely vascularised. The corneal grafts in this

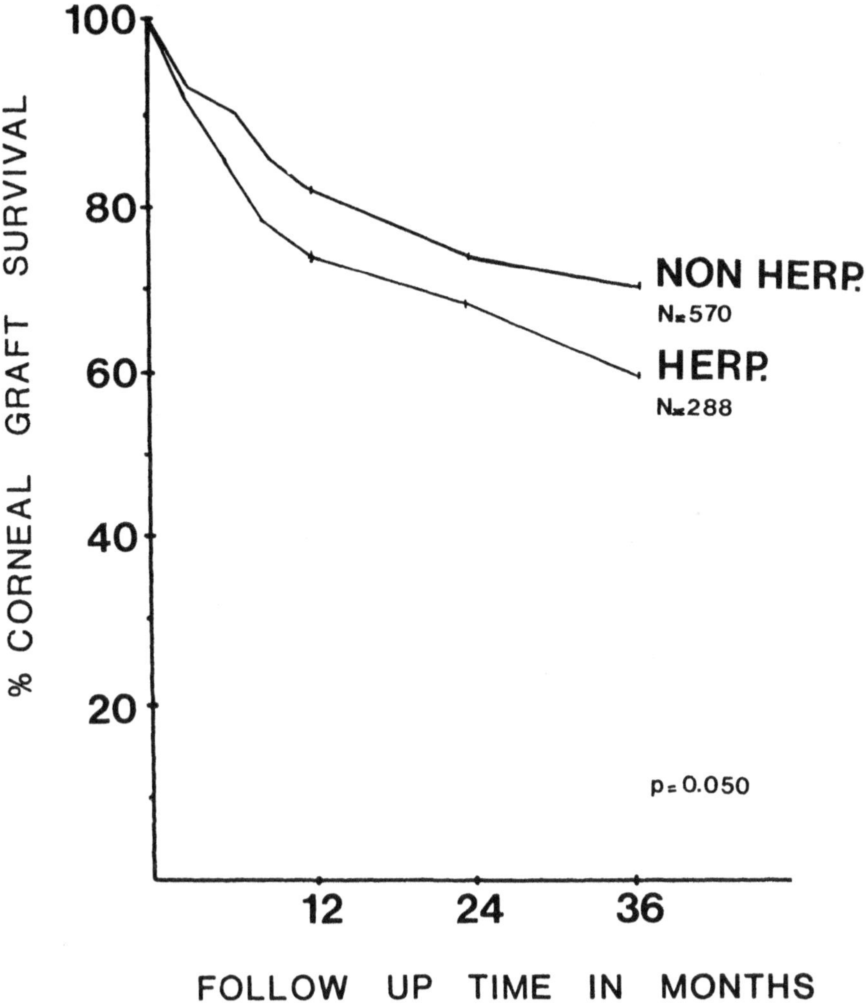

Figure 1. Corneal graft survival in eyes grafted because of recurrent herpes simplex virus keratitis versus non herpetic eye diseases.

group of patients demonstrated a lower, but not significantly lower, survival as compared to the remaining 224 vascularised corneas; 68.2%, 58.4% and 36.7% versus 73.1%, 66.1% and 57.7% at one, two and three years (fig. not shown).

Apart from the recurrence of HSV keratitis in the grafts for HSV keratitis, the causes of graft failures (rejection, glaucoma, infection, trauma) are not significantly different when compared to the causes of graft failure in corneal grafts for non-herpetic diseases. Since herpetic infection may induce graft rejection, it is difficult to determine whether or not grafts became opaque

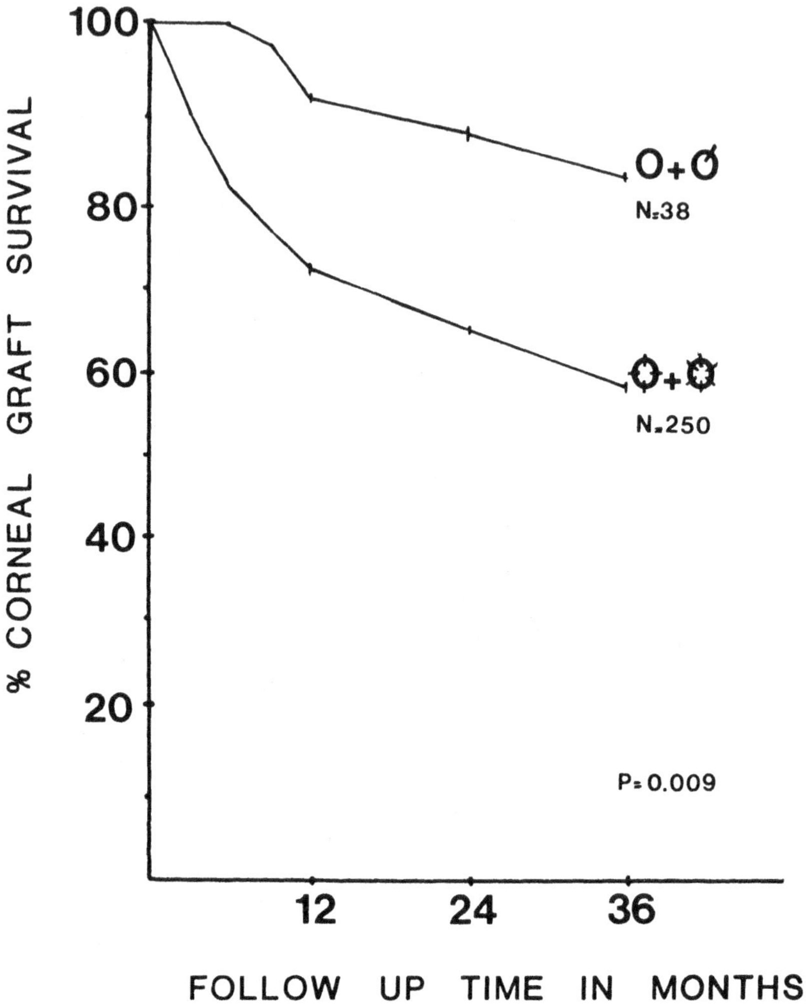

Figure 2. Influence of vascularisation on corneal graft survival
O = no vessel ingrowth — = moderately vascularised
ϕ = slightly vascularised — = severely vascularised

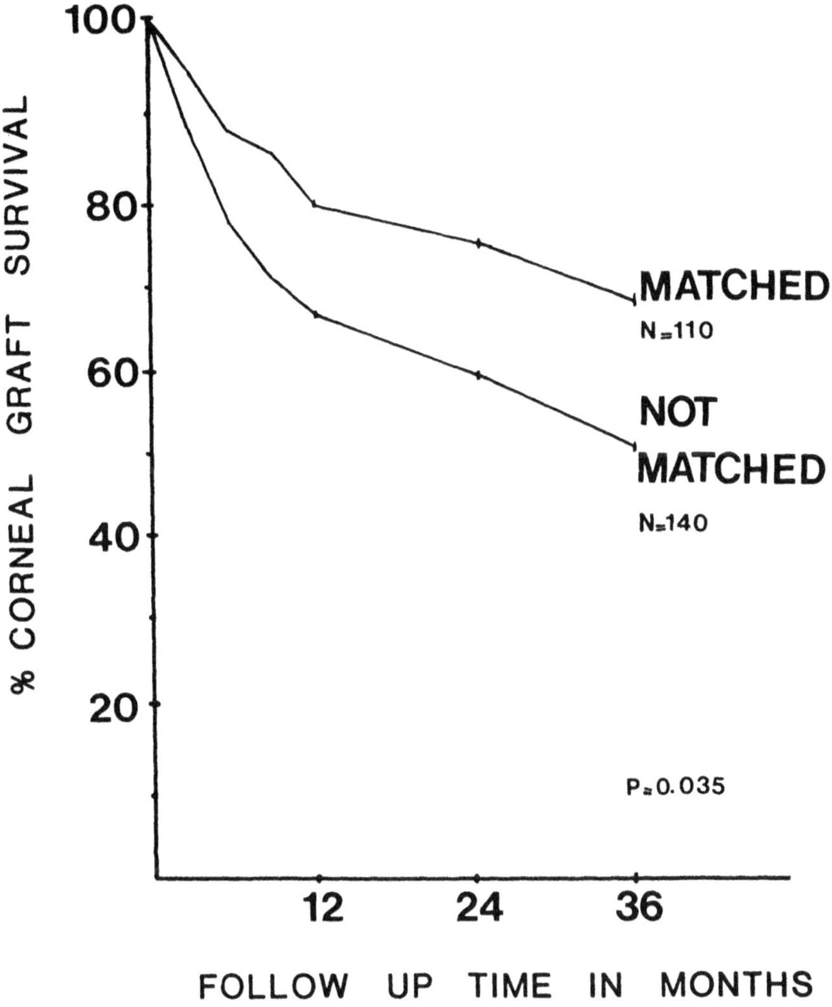

Figure 3. The effect of prospectively HLA-A and -B matching on corneal graft survival in vascularised corneas with recurrent herpes simplex virus keratitis.

because of HSV infections or because of rejection (Rice and Jones 1973). Although not every HSV infection causes a graft rejection, they remain a potential danger.

In the 288 corneal grafts for recurrent HSV keratitis, a recurrence of the HSV in the graft was observed in 42 cases (See colour plate 8, a and b). In 15 of them, the graft became opaque subsequently. The percentage of herpetic recurrences in the first year after keratoplasty was 9.4% (17 recurrences of HSV and 181 patients at risk for 12 months), 10.2% in the second year (13 recurrences of HSV and 128 patients at risk for 24 months) and 11.0% in the

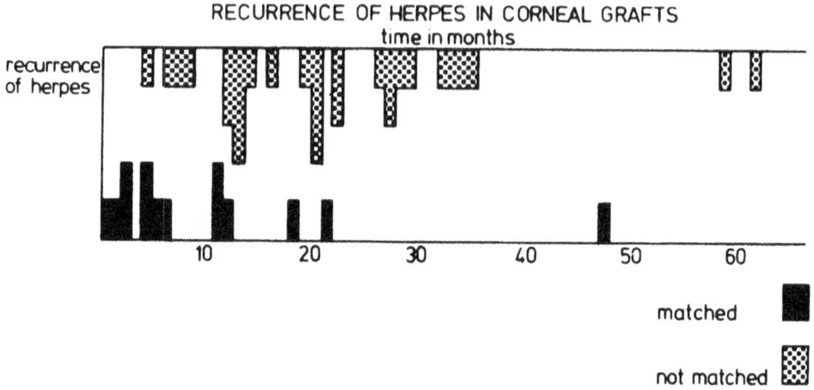

Figure 4. Time interval between penetrating keratoplasty and the recurrence of herpes simplex virus in HLA-A and -B matched grafts as compared with not matched grafts (p = 0.0004).

third year (9 recurrences of HSV and 82 patients at risk for 36 months). The time lapse between PKP and the recurrence of HSV in the grafts varied from less than one month to 62 months (fig. 4). A highly significant shorter interval between PKP and recurrence of HSV in the graft was observed in HLA-A and -B matched grafts as compared to unmatched grafts: 8.0 months for the matched grafts and 19.4 months for the unmatched grafts; Mann Whitney U test, p=0.0004).

Discussion

The results of the penetrating keratoplasties in herpes simplex virus keratitis are described by several authors (Beekhuis et al. 1983, Cobo et al. 1980, Fine et al. 1977, Foster et al. 1981 and Polack et al. 1972). Cobo was the only one who used the actuarial life table method to evaluate the survival of 132 grafts in his study. He observed a survival of 72% at one year and 64% at two and three years. This is comparable to our results of 73.0%, 68.2% and 60.4% graft survival at one, two and three years in our entire group of 288 transplants. Cobo reported also a graft survival rate of 44% at two years in 33 eyes which were actively inflamed at the time of surgery. This suggests that they may have been transplanted à chaud. His results are comparable to our observation of 58.4% clear grafts at two years in 26 transplants performed à chaud. Cobo's observation that pre- operative vascularisation is the major prognostic factor was previously described by Batchelor et al. (1976), confirmed by us in 1982 and in this study (p=0.009). Neither in Cobo's study nor in ours was a significant difference in herpetic recurrence found between the group of clinically non-inflamed eyes versus actively inflamed eyes at the time of graft surgery. This observation is not surprising since it was demonstrated by means of electron microscopy that viral particles were present in a corneal button removed at the time of transplantation in an eye which was clinically non-inflamed during 1.5 years pre- operatively (fig. 5) (Van de Want 1980).

Beekhuis et al. studied 23 patients with active herpetic corneal disease and 23 patients with clinically inactive corneal disease at the time of transplantation. Although they did not use the life table method to evaluate the percentage of clear grafts, they did follow up all their patients for a minimum of 5 years. Unfortunately both patient groups in their study consisted of lamellar grafts as well as full thickness grafts. The prognosis of lamellar grafts is poorer than for full thickness grafts (Rice et al. 1973). Therefore, we cannot compare their results with ours.

It was not possible to determine if there was any agreement between the results reported by Fine et al. (1977), Foster et al. (1981) and Polack et al.

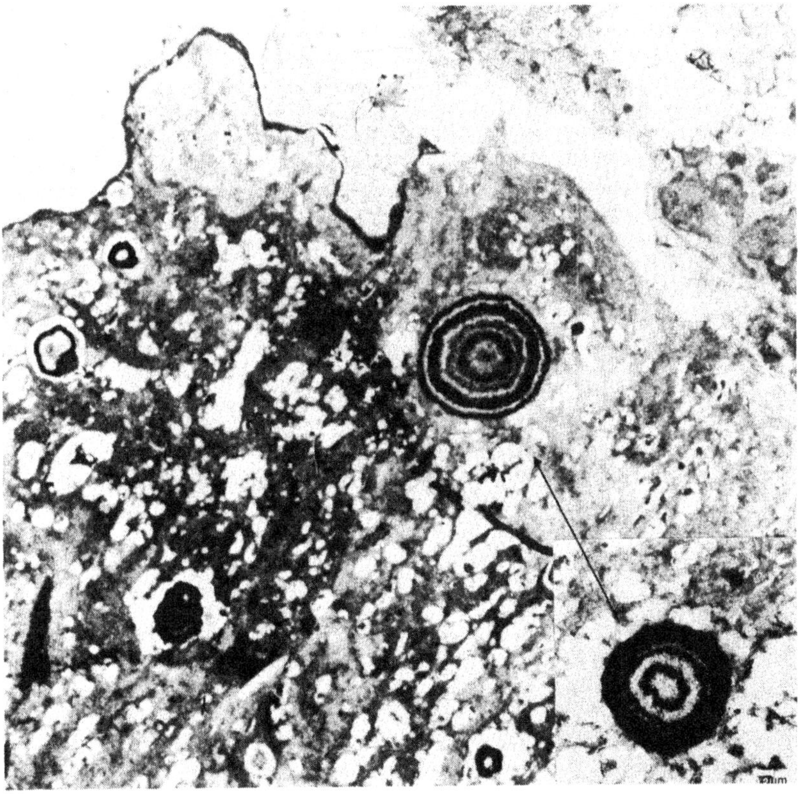

Figure 5. Electron micrographe of herpes simplex virus particle in the corneal stroma of a corneal button removed at the time of graft surgery in an eye which was clinically non inflamed during 1.5 years preoperatively (magn. 25.000x).

(1972) and ours because the method used to evaluate the percentage of clear grafts was not appropriate to the data. An actuarial life table method as used by Cobo et al. (1980) and in our study is the only valid method for such data since patients are entering the study at different periods and are followed up for different lengths of time (Peto, et al. 1976).

The effect of HLA-A and -B matching on corneal graft survival in grafts performed because ofrecurrent HSV keratitis has to our knowledge not yet been described. We observed two effects. Firstly, a significant beneficial effect (p=0.035) of HLA-A and -B matching on corneal graft survival in vascularised corneas with recurrent HSV keratitis. This observation confirms our previous observation of a significantly increased graft survival with the use of prospectively matched donor corneas in vascularised corneas, independent of the initial indication for grafting (chapter 6). Secondly, there is a significant decrease in the time interval between PKP and recurrence of HSV in the matched grafts, as compared to the unmatched graft (p=0.0004). Since the HSV is a neurotrophical virus, the reinnervation rate of the denervated donor cornea button may influence the recurrence of HSV. Corneal sensibility, as a parameter for corneal nerve ingrowth, can be measured with a corneal aesthesiometer (Skriver 1978, Draeger et al. 1979). We could not demonstrate corneal sensibility in the first year after grafting in a group of 16 corneas grafted because of recurrent HSV. However, we have observed a measurable corneal sensibility in 4 of the 7 HLA-A and -B matched grafts while only one of the 9 unmatched grafts demonstrated a measurable corneal sensibility 19 months after keratoplasty (Kok-van Alphen et al. 1983). Those results suggest that nerve ingrowth in an HLA matched graft is faster than in unmatched grafts. Consequently, it is not surprising that recurrences of the HSV are observed in an earlier postoperative period in the well matched group. Although the earlier recurrences of the HSV may induce a rejection episode in a more 'dangerous' period after grafting, it is apparent that the positive influence of HLA matching overrules the possible negative influence of early HSV recurrences.

During the past ten years several studies (Cobo et al. 1980, Colin et al. 1978, Foster et al. 1981, Pouliquen et al. 1981, Pfister et al. 1972, Witmer 1981 and Sie 1980) on the recurrence of HSV after keratoplasty have been reported. The rate of recurrence of HSV varied from 8% to 75%. The follow up times varied from one to 15 years. The HSV recurrence rate seems to increase with time (Cobo et al. 1980 and Foster et al. 1981) while Sie (1980) reported in a review of the literature that the majority of the HSV recurrences are observed in the first year after grafting. In our material, we observed almost the same percentage of herpes recurrences in the first, the second and the third year (9.4%, 10.2% and 11.0%) so. we do not confirm the observations reported by Cobo, Foster and Sie. It was difficult to determine whether or not Cobo and Foster had calculated the percentage of herpes recurrence by dividing the number of HSV recurrences by the number of patients 'at risk' at one, two or three years. In most of the studies the total number of HSV recurrences is divided by the total number of patients at the start of the study instead of the number of patients that had been followed up for one, two or three years respectively.

Conclusion

The use of keratoplasty as the therapy for herpetic keratitis is applied in the vast majority of cases, to corneas with severe vessel ingrowth. The success of penetrating keratoplasties is inversely proportional to the degree of the corneal vascularisation ($p=0.009$). We were able to improve our results with the use of HLA-A and -B matched grafts; a significantly better graft survival was observed in matched grafts when compared to unmatched grafts ($p=0.035$). HLA-A and -B matched grafts demonstrated a significantly decreased time lapse between keratoplasty and the recurrence of herpetic simplex in the graft as compared to unmatched grafts ($p=0.0004$). The majority of the herpetic recurrences in the matched grafts were observed in the first post operative year while the unmatched grafts demonstrated the majority of the herpetic recurrences in the second post operative year. Two thirds of all herpetic recurrences in the graft healed without signs of opacification. We consider it advisable to use HLA-A and -B matched donor material when grafting vascularised corneas with herpetic keratitis. These patients should be kept under regular ophthalmological observation, especially in the first postoperative year.

References

Batchelor J.R., Casey T.A, Gibbs D.C., Loyd D.F., Werb A, Prasad S.S. and James A. (1976) HLA matching and corneal grafting. The Lancet 1: 551-554.

Beekhuis W.H., Renardel de Lavalette J.G.C., Van Rij G. and Schaap G.J.P. (1983) Therapeutic keratoplasty for active herpetic corneal disease; viral culture and prognosis. Documenta Ophthalmol. 55: 31-35.

Cobo L.M., Coster D.J., Rice N.S.C., Jones B.R. (1980) Prognosis and management of corneal transplantation for herpetic keratitis. Arch. Ophthalmol. 98: 1755-1759.

Colin J., Goichot E.L. and Petroutsos G. (1981) Complications des kératoplasties sur kératitite herpétiques. J.Fr.Ophthalmol. 4: 12, 829-832.

Draeger J., Koudelka A. and Lubahn E. (1976) Zur Aesthesiometrie der Hornhaut. Klin. med. Augenheilk. 169: 407-421.

Fine N, Cignetti F.E. (1977) Penetrating keratoplasty in herpes simplex keratitis recurrence in grafts. Arch. Ophthalmol. 95: 613-616.

Foster C. (1981) Penetrating keratoplasty for herpes simplex keratitis. In: Sundmacher R, (Hrsg) Herpetic Eye Diseases, Munich, Bergmann, p 425.

Harms H, Mackensen H. (1966) Augenoperationen unter dem Mikroskop. p. 291. Thieme Verlag, Stuttgart.

Kok-van Alphen C.C., Völker-Dieben H.J., Graniewsky-Wijnands H. (1983) Cornea aesthesiometry after perforating keratoplasty. In press.

Peto R., Pike M.C, Armitage P., Breslow N.E., Cox D.R., Howard S.V., Mantel N., McPherson K., Peto J., Smith P.G. (1976) Design and analysis of randomized clinical trials requiring prolonged observation of each patient. Br.J. Cancer 34: 585.

Pfister R.R., Richards J.S.F., Dohlman C.H. (1972) Recurrence of herpetic keratitis in corneal grafts. Am.J.Ophthalmol. 73: 192-196.

Polack F.P., Kaufman H.E. (1972) Penetrating keratoplasty in herpetic keratitis. Am.J.Ophthal. 73: 908-913.

Pouliquen J., Goichot E.L., Petroutsos G. (1981) Complications des kéroplasties sur kératitite herpétiques. J.Fr.Ophthalmol. 4: 12, 829-832.

Rice N.S.C. and Jones B.R. Problems of corneal grafting in herpetic keratitis. (1973) Ciba Foundation Symposium on Corneal Graft Failure. Amsterdam, Associated Scientific Publication, 15: p. 221-239.

Sie S.H. (1980) Recidivprophylaxe mit Trifluorothymidin nach Keratoplastik bei Herpes corneae. Ophthalmologica, Basel 180: 1-8.

Skriver K. (1978) Reinnervation of the corneal graft. Acta Ophthalmologica 56: 1013-1015.

Want v.d. H. (1980) Personal communication.

Witmer R. (1981) Results of keratoplasty in meta herpetic keratitis. In: Sudmacher R, (Hrsg). Herpetic Eye Diseases, Munich, Bergmann, p 419

SECTION III

HLA and ABO associations in eye diseases

CHAPTER 11

HLA-A and -B antigens in recurrent corneal herpes simplex virus infection*

Summary

115 Patients with recurrent herpetic keratitis and 123 controls were studied for the distribution of HLA-A, -B and -C antigens. HLA-A3 was found to be significantly more frequent in the herpes population (corrected p value = 0.042). Also, males were nearly twice as frequently affected as females ($p<0.001$). Females seem to be less susceptible for HSV keratitis between the ages of 15 to 45.

Introduction

The human histocompatibility complex, HLA, plays an important role in immune responsiveness and in susceptibility to disease and its subsequent clinical course (Van Rood 1980). Two reports on the association of HLA and recurrent Herpes Simplex Virus (HSV) infection have been published. Zimmerman et al. (1977) reported an increased frequency of HLA-B5 in recurrent HSV keratitis. Meyers-Elliott et al. (1980) reported that HLA-Aw30 occurred three times more frequently in patients with HSV keratitis than in normal whites. However, these p values were not significant after correction.

The almost universal human infection by HSV makes it all the more remarkable that corneal HSV infection is relatively rare. Corneal HSV keratitis is not a very serious infection in its initial phase. The recurrent version develops in 25% of the cases and the eventual condition of the cornea may become so bad that corneal transplantation is indicated. One third of our corneal transplantion patients have the diagnosis of recurrent HSV keratitis.

Subjects and methods

Patients (N=115) and healthy controls (N=123) were all selected from the Dutch population in order to avoid spurious associations due to ethnic

* *For colour plates, see pp. 72ff.*

differences or mixtures. The HLA antigens of the 115 patients were analysed for a possible association between the HLA-A, -B and -C antigens and the predisposition to recurrent HSV keratitis.

Typing for 8 HLA-A, 16 HLA-B and 6 HLA-C antigens was performed by using the microlymphocytotoxicity test (Van Rood 1979). The HLA frequencies of the patients were compared to those of a control group of 123 normal persons typed in the same laboratory in Leyden. The Woolf-Haldane (1955) analysis was used to assess the significance of the different antigen frequencies in these patients and controls. All p values were corrected for a total of 30 antigens studied using the procedure suggested by Edwards (1974).

Results

HLA and disease association

The HLA-A phenotype frequencies for the patients with recurrent HSV keratitis and the controls are shown in table 1. HLA-A3 was found to be significantly increased, the corrected p value = 0.042. There were no significant differences in any of the other HLA antigen frequencies.

The HLA-B and HLA-C phenotype frequencies for the patients and controls are shown in tables 2 and 3. There were no significantly increased frequencies for the HLA-B or HLA-C antigens.

Sex ratio in recurrent HSV keratitis

We found a striking sex difference. In 131 patients with recurrent HSV keratitis (of which 115 were HLA typed) we found almost two times more males than females, i.e. 85 male patients and 46 females. This differential sex distribution was highly significant (chi square = 11.61, $p<0.001$).

Table 1. Woolf-Haldane analysis of the HLA-A antigen frequencies in 115 patients with recurrent corneal herpes and in 123 healthy controls

Antigen	Patients pos.	neg.	Controls pos.	neg.	Relative risk	Chi. square	p corr.*
A1	34	81	41	82	0.842	0.389	n.s.
A2	54	61	63	60	0.844	0.432	n.s.
A3	45	70	24	99	2.621	10.819	0.042
A9	21	94	24	99	0.924	0.059	n.s.
A10	2	113	12	111	0.196	6.187	n.s.
A11	8	107	18	105	0.451	3.477	n.s.
A28	16	99	10	113	1.793	2.021	n.s.
Aw19	24	91	28	95	0.897	0.123	n.s.

* p values have been corrected for a total of 30 comparisons n.s. = not significant

Table 2. Woolf-Haldane analysis of the HLA-B antigen frequencies in 115 patients with recurrent corneal herpes and in 123 healty controls

Antigen	Patients		Controls		Relative	Chi.	p
	pos.	neg.	pos.	neg.	risk	square	corr.*
B5	17	98	20	103	0.984	0.002	n.s.
B7	27	88	20	103	1.720	2.849	n.s.
B8	36	79	29	94	1.471	1.785	n.s.
B12	26	89	28	95	0.992	0.001	n.s.
B13	6	109	6	117	1.073	0.016	n.s.
B14	3	112	2	121	1.512	0.285	n.s.
B15	16	99	16	107	1.080	0.044	n.s.
Bw16	13	102	10	113	1.424	0.690	n.s.
B17	7	108	12	111	0.617	1.063	n.s.
B18	7	108	15	108	0.484	2.560	n.s.
Bw21	4	111	7	116	0.627	0.637	n.s.
Bw22	2	113	10	113	0.238	4.662	n.s.
B27	10	105	13	110	0.815	0.232	n.s.
Bw35	18	97	20	103	0.958	0.015	n.s.
B37	1	114	4	119	0.348	1.555	n.s.
B40	20	95	15	108	1.503	1.278	n.s.

* p values have been corrected for a total of 30 comparisons n.s. = not significant

Table 3. Woolf-Haldane analysis of the HLA-C antigen frequencies in 115 patients with recurrent corneal herpes and in 123 healthy controls

Antigen	Patients		Controls		Relative	Chi.	p
	pos.	neg.	pos.	neg.	risk	square	corr.*
C21	5	110	11	112	0.487	1.934	n.s.
Cw2	14	101	12	111	1.274	0.362	n.s.
Cw3	35	80	29	94	1.413	1.421	n.s.
Cw4	22	93	22	101	1.086	0.063	n.s.
Cw5	10	82	11	112	1.245	0.246	n.s.
Cw6	10	49	26	97	0.780	0.389	n.s.

* p values have been corrected for a total of 30 comparisons. n.s. = not significant

The ages of onset of the primary HSV infection are shown in fig. 1. It was found that 56% of the male patients incurred their primary HSV infection between the ages of 15 and 45 years. Only 26% of the female patients incurred their primary infection in that age span.

Duration of the recurrent HSV keratitis

The 131 patients with recurrent HSV keratitis were all grafted in the corneal department of the Leyden University Hospital. The average duration of the recurrent HSV keratitis was 17.7 years (2-65 years) at the time of transplantation. The age of the patients varied from 5 to 81 years, average 51.2 years.

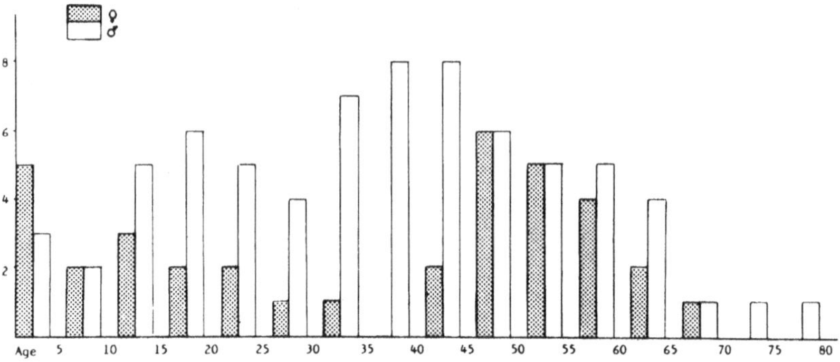

Figure 1. Ages of onset of the primary HSV infection

Discussion

Our findings of a significantly increased frequency of HLA-A3 in 115 patients with recurrent HSV keratitis when compared to their controls (corr. p value = 0.042) does not agree with the findings of Zimmerman et al. (1977) who studied 46 patients, nor with the findings of Meyers-Elliott et al. (1980) who studied 48 patients.

Zimmerman et al. (1977) reported an increased frequency of HLA-B5 in 46 patients with recurrent corneal HSV as compared to 282 normal controls. However, the increase is not significant when the p value is corrected for the 32 antigens which were studied. In addition, there is uncertainty about the patient and control populations which are referred only as 'white' and 'normal' respectively. Even if the subjects were all Caucasoids, that would not exclude population heterogeneity and it could be the reason for the differential antigen frequencies in patients and controls.

Meyers-Elliott et al. (1980) reported an HLA-Aw30 increased frequency but this was not significant after correction. Incidentally, these authors corrected the p value only for the 14 antigens in the HLA-A locus instead of for the total 40 antigens in the HLA-A, -B and -C and -DR loci. If they had done so, they would have obtained a corrected p value of 1.20 using the method which they cited. The proper correction is $1\text{-}(1\text{-}0.3)^{40} = 0.70$. Finally a precise description of the populations is not found in their report. They speak of patients and normal whites. Therefore, as in the Zimmerman report, we are confronted again with the possibility of population heterogeneity as a possible explanation for the differential antigen frequencies in patients and controls.

The highly significant difference in the numbers of male and female patients (85 male, 46 female) with recurrent HSV keratitis, and the fact that 56% of the male patients as compared to 26% of the female patients incurred their primary HSV infection between the ages of 15 and 45 years, cannot be explained at this time. One possibility is that females between 15 and 45 demonstrate a beneficial effect of hormonal factors during their reproductive period. Further studies are necessary to test this hypothesis.

Conclusion

- HLA-A, -B and -C typing of patients with recurrent HSV keratitis revealed a significantly increased frequency of HLA-A3 (corrected p=0.042).
- Almost twice as many male patients (N=85) as female(N=46) were found in the group of patients with recurrent HSV keratitis. This differential sexdistribution was highly significant (p 0.001.)
- Female patients seem to be less susceptible for the HSV keratitis between the age of 15 to 45.
- Using matched homogenous patients and control population would facilitate the comparisons of findings in different studies.

References

Edwards J.H. (1974) HLA and disease. The detection of associations. J. Immunogenet. 1: 249.

Haldane J.B.S. (1955) The estimation and signficance of the logarithm of a ratio of frequencies. Ann. Hum. Genet. 20: 30.

Meyers-Elliott R.H. et al. (1980) HLA antigens in herpes stromal keratitis. Am. Ophthalmol. 89: 54-58.

Rood Van J.J. (1979) Microlymphocytotoxicity method. In: NIAID Manual of tissue typing techniques (Ed: (J. Ray) National Institute of Health (NIH) (80-545) Maryland, U.S.A.: 104.

Rood Van J.J. (1980) The genetics and biology of the HLA system. In: Benacerraf B., Dorf M.E. (eds) The role of the major histocompatibility complex in immunology. Garland, New York.

Woolf B. (1955) On estimating the relation between blood groups and disease. Ann. Hum. Genet. 19: 251.

Zimmerman T.J. et al. (1977) HLA type and recurrent corneal herpes simplex infection. Invest. Ophthalmol. Visual Sci. 15: 756.

CHAPTER 12

HLA-DR antigens in recurrent corneal herpes simplex virus infection*

The relative rarity of Herpes Simplex Virus (HSV) eye infections, when compared to the wide diffusion of general HSV infection (Leopold and Sery 1963), prompted us to look for HLA antigen associations and susceptibility for the disease. In chapter 11 we have reported on HLA-A, -B and -C antigen associations and HSV keratitis. In this study we have looked for HLA-DR antigen associations and susceptibility for HSV keratitis.

HLA-DR typings were performed on 28 patients, 17 males and 11 females, who were grafted because of severe recurrent herpes simplex virus (HSV) keratitis. The diagnosis of herpes simplex keratitis was made clinically since negative virus cultures do not rule out that diagnosis in longstanding cases. By means of electronmicroscopy, it was possible to demonstrate viral particles in the excised corneal button of one patient (chapter 10) who had a negative culture, but this technique was not routinely applied. The frequencies of the antigens in the patients were compared to those of 200 healthy non related persons. All of the patients and controls were of Dutch Caucasoid origin. Analysis and statistical methods used were as previously described (Völker-Dieben et al. 1983).

The only antigen with a significantly different frequency before correction for the number of antigens studied was HLA-DRw8, RR=8.203, X^2=10.501, p=0.002, see table 1. We corrected the p value for 40 antigens the 10 DR antigens in this study and the 30 A, B and C antigens in our previous study (chapter 11). It is noteworthy that three out of four patients with HLA-DRw8 were also positive for A2 and B5. There is no significant linkage disequilibrium between A2 and B5 or between B5 and DRw8 in the Dutch Caucasoid population.

Our results do not confirm the elevated frequency of HLA-DRw7, not significant after correction, in 34 patients with recurrent HSV keratitis reported by Meyers-Elliot et al. (1980). Those authors did not report any data for DRw8, DRw9 and DRw10 so that our observation of a significantly elevated frequency of DRw8 before correction must await confirmation in future studies. Finally, the excess of males among our patients is consistent with our previous report of a highly significant excess of male over female patients with herpes simplex virus keratitis (chapter 11).

* *For colour plates, see pp. 72ff.*

Table 1. HLA-DR antigen frequencies in 28 patients with recurrent herpes simplex virus keratitis and in 200 healthy controls

Antigen	Patients pos.	neg.	Controls pos.	neg.	Relative risk	Chi. square	p value
DR1	5	18	41	159	1.143	0.071	n.s.
DR2	3	20	54	146	0.459	1.880	n.s.
DR3	6	17	57	142	0.920	0.031	n.s.
DR4	9	14	49	151	2.005	2.505	n.s.
DR5	3	20	46	153	0.564	1.010	n.s.
DRw6	6	17	58	142	0.905	0.045	n.s.
DR7	7	16	50	150	1.355	0.439	n.s.
DRw8	4	19	5	195	8.203	10.501	0.002*
DRw9	0	22	6	193	0.662	0.143	n.s.
DRw10	2	21	10	190	2.110	1.173	n.s.

* p value significant before correction for the total of 40 HLA antigens examined in this study and in our previous study of HLA-A, -B and -C (chapter 11)

n.s. = not significant

REFERENCES

Leopold I.H. and Sery T.W. (1963) Epidemiology of herpes simplex keratitis. Invest. Ophthalmol. Visual Sci. 2: 298.

Meyers-Elliott, R.H., Maxwell, W.H. and Petit, T.H. (1981) HLA-DR and susceptibility to Recurrent Herpes Simplex Stromal Keratitis and Progenitalis. In Herpetische Augenerkrankungen, J.F. Bergman Verlag, München, p. 81.

Völker-Dieben, H.J.M., D'Amaro, J., De Lange, P. and Wolff-Rouendaal, D. (1983) HLA and ABO antigens in malignant choroidal melanoma. Clin. Exp. Immunol. 53: 581-588.

CHAPTER 13

HLA and ABO antigens in keratoconus patients*

Summary

Fourty-two patients with a keratoconus and 200 controls were studied for the distribution of HLA-A, -B and -C antigens. No significant HLA-A, -B and -C associations were observed. The excess of males in our patient population, although not significant, confirmed similar findings by three other investigators.

Introduction

Keratoconus is an axial ectasia of the cornea, usually bilateral, which manifests itself after the onset of puberty (See fig. 1). It is a hereditary disorder, but sporadic cases occur frequently. The central cornea becomes thin and Bowman's layer is destroyed in most cases. Acute hydrops may occur due to ruptures of Descemet's membrane (Grayson et al. 1979). Visual acuity becomes severely reduced either due to the frequently uncorrectable irregular corneal astigmatism, or the corneal oedema, and later by scar formation of the cornea after the acute hydrops. The only effective treatment is penetrating keratoplasty. 42 Patients with a keratoconus were tissue typed to enable us to match them with their corneal donors. Since keratoconus has a hereditary component, we decided to analyse HLA-A, -B and -C antigen frequencies in those patients.

Material and methods

Fourty-two Dutch patients and 200 healthy unrelated Dutch controls of Caucasoid origin were the subject of this study. Typing for 8 HLA-A, 16 HLA-B and 6 HLA-C antigens and the statistical methods were as previously described. (Völker-Dieben et al. 1983).

In all keratoconus patients, 26 male patients and 16 females, the corneal buttons excised at the time of keratoplasty were histologically examined, and the clinical diagnosis was confirmed in all cases. The ages of the patients ranged from 10 to 68 years, average 36.7 years.

* *For colour plates, see pp. 72ff.*

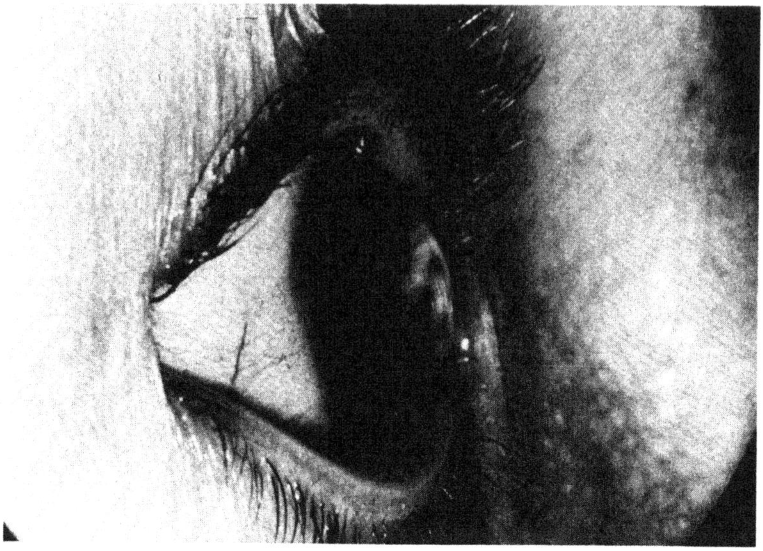

Figure 1. Severe keratoconus.

Results

HLA Associations

In 42 patients with keratoconus no significant HLA associations were observed (table 1). There were 3 antigens which were never positive in those patients (B16, Bw21 and B37) with chances of occurring at least once in that patient population of 95%, 47% and 78% respectively.

ABO Bloodgroups

The distribution of the ABO bloodgroups in the total patient group (table 2) was not significantly different from that of the Dutch control population (Nijenhuis, 1961).

Sex distribution

There are relatively more male patients (N=26) than female patients (N=16) in this keratoconus patient group but the male to female distribution is not significantly different from a 1:1 ratio.

Table 1. Woolf-Haldane analysis of the HLA antigen frequencies in 42 keratoconus patients and controls

Antigen	Patients pos.	Patients neg.	Controls pos.	Controls neg.	Relative risk	Chi. square	p value
A1	13	29	68	132	0.885	0.117	0.730
A2	24	18	105	95	1.199	0.292	0.596
A3	9	33	51	149	0.823	0.244	0.628
A9	10	32	39	161	1.321	0.508	0.483
A10	2	40	7	193	1.593	0.444	0.513
A11	3	39	25	175	0.610	0.766	0.385
A28	5	37	17	183	1.538	0.729	0.398
Aw19	9	33	46	154	0.942	0.023	0.853
B5	6	36	24	176	1.283	0.288	0.598
B7	10	32	51	149	0.938	0.028	0.843
B8	13	29	45	155	1.564	1.505	0.218
B12	16	26	60	140	1.446	1.140	0.286
B13	2	40	6	194	1.847	0.745	0.393
B14	3	39	8	192	2.007	1.240	0.265
B15	9	33	31	169	1.526	1.072	0.301
Bw16	0	42	14	186	0.151	3.256	0.068
B17	1	41	20	180	0.318	2.272	0.128
B18	1	41	15	185	0.433	1.187	0.276
Bw21	0	42	3	107	0.664	0.131	0.716
Bw22	2	40	9	191	1.244	0.103	0.744
B27	2	40	15	185	0.739	0.215	0.648
Bw35	6	36	35	165	0.830	0.170	0.683
B37	0	42	7	193	0.304	1.232	0.266
B40	9	33	25	175	1.952	2.577	0.104
Cw1	4	38	7	193	3.016	3.424	0.061
Cw2	3	39	17	182	0.924	0.019	0.862
Cw3	16	26	62	137	1.370	0.832	0.365
Cw4	10	32	39	159	1.305	0.464	0.503
Cw5	3	31	30	165	0.603	0.801	0.374
Cw6	2	27	26	154	0.530	0.977	0.324

Discussion

An overview of the HLA-antigen association studies in patients with keratoconus and their results are set out in table 3.

The lack of significantly increased HLA antigen associations in

Table 2. ABO blood groups in 42 keratoconus patients

	N	blood groups O	A	B	AB
Male	26	10	12	2	2
Female	16	9	7	0	0
Total	42	19	19	2	2

Table 3. An overview of HLA Antigen association studies in patients with keratoconsus

Author	Number of Patients	Antigens	Land of origin
Gasset et al. 1977	4	B27	Florida
Vannas et al. 1977	56	no deviation	Finland
	(7)*	(B12 and B27)*	Finland
Damgaard-Jensen et al. 1979	42	B7	Denmark
	40	B15	
Karantinos et al. 1980	20	Bw21	Greece
Blagojevic et al. 1980	27	A9	Yugoslavia
		A10	
		B12	
Wachtmeister et al. 1982	30	no deviation	Sweden
Klouda et al. 1983	64	B5	Great Britain
Völker-Dieben et al. (this study)	42	no deviation	The Netherlands

* In 7 patients with a corneal graft rejection HLA-B12 and B27 were elevated.

keratoconus patients in our study does not agree with the results of Damgaard-Jansen et al. (1979) who also studied 42 patients, Karantinos et al. (1980) who studied 20 patients, Blagojevic et al. (1980) who studied 27 patients and Klouda et al. (1983) who studied 64 patients, but it confirms the observation of Vannas et al. (1977) and Wachtmeister et al. (1982), who also did not find any significant antigen deviations (table 3).

Karantinos et al. (1980) diagnosed keratoconus on the basis of clinical examinations including keratometer readings, refraction, photodiagnosis and biomicroscopy. They reported an increased frequency of Bw21 in 20 keratoconus patients ($p=0.001$). His patient population was referred to as Caucasian Greek persons and his controls as 200 healthy persons from the Greek population. After correction for the total number of antigens studied $(1-(1-0.001)^{26}$, the p value was still significant. None of the patients in our study were positive for Bw21. However, the absence of Bw16 in our patients is confirmed in their patients.

Blagojevic et al. (1980) reported an increased frequency of A9, A10 and B12 antigens ($p<0.05$). His patient population was composed of patients attending the Contact lens Department. It was not clear if these patients are unrelated persons. His control population is referred to as 122 healthy unrelated persons. Even if the subjects were all Caucasoids that would not exclude population heterogeneity (D'Amaro et al., 1983). Furthermore, the diagnosis of keratoconus was not based on histological examinations. Since keratoconus is usually a bilateral condition, we were surprised by the high number (10 out of the 27 patients) of unilateral cases reported by Blagojevic et al. (1980).

The diagnosis of keratoconus is not always easy to make, as illustrated by fig. 2. which shows the histology of a corneal button excised at the time of transplantation from a patient not included in our study. This 31 year old woman was diagnosed by us clinically as a keratoconus patient. Severe

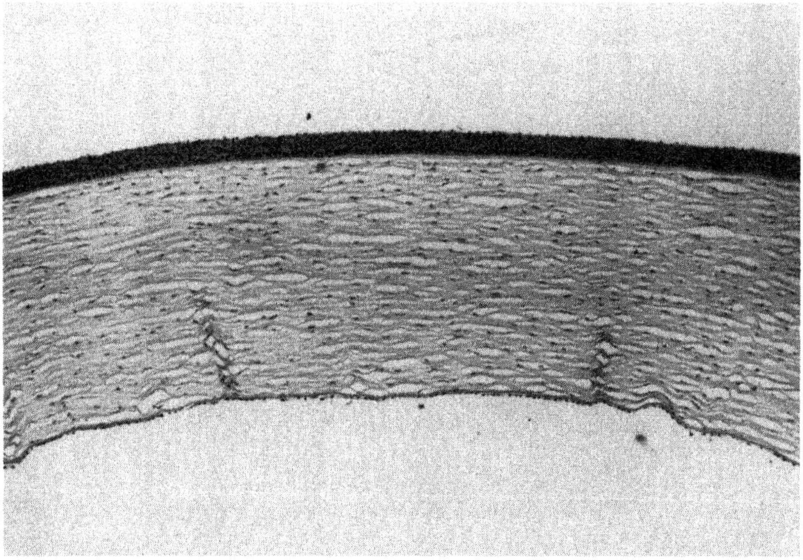

Figure 2. Corneal button excised, at the time of transplantation, from a 31 year old woman. Astigmatism was over 9 Diopters, irregular. A clinical diagnosis of keratoconus was made, however histologic examination ruled it out. The epithelial layer is regular. Bowmans' layer is intact, i.e. there are not breaks through which keratocyte or collagen fibers can push towards the epithelium. There is no evidence for (healed) ruptures in Descemets' membrane (Magnification 64×).

astigmatism was observed in both eyes. In the eye which was later grafted, the astigmatism was over 9 Diopters and irregular. Contact lenses were not tolerated anymore. Histologic examination (by M. Gorsira) ruled out the diagnosis of keratoconus.

Klouda et al. (1983) investigated the HLA-A and -B phenotypes in 64 Caucasoid patients from South West England. Their clinical criteria for the diagnosis included keratometer readings and slitlamp findings. Histological examinations were not mentioned. They observed a significant increase of B5 (p corr.=0.01).

The 30 keratoconus patients studied by Wachtmeister et al. (1982) were also clinically diagnosed and no histological examinations were mentioned. Their precise diagnostic criteria are mentioned in their report. Patients and controls are referred to as unrelated Caucasians. They observed no significant deviations in the frequencies of the HLA-A and B antigens. Our results, therefore are consistent with their findings. HLA-Bw16 was found twice in their patient group while we did not observe this antigen in our patients. The observation of Vannas et al. (1977) that HLA-B12 and HLA-B27 are increased in the keratoconus patients who rejected their corneal allografts was not observed in the 6 patients in our study who rejected their grafts.

The excess of males in our patient group (26 males and 16 females) is not significantly different from the distribution in the patients groups of Karantinos et al. (1980), Blagojevic et al. (1980) and Wachtmeister et al. (1982) (table 4).

Table 4. Sex distribution in 42 keratoconus patients

	Males	Females
Karantinos et al. 1980	14	6
Blagojevic et al. 1980	18	9
Wachtmeister et al. 1982	27	3
Völker-Dieben et al. (this study)	26	16

$X^2 = 7.257$, degrees of freedom 3, $p = 0.06$

Conclusions

- No significant HLA-A, -B and -C associations were observed in a group of 42 keratoconus patients.
- HLA-Bw16 was never observed in this patient group although the chance of observing one positive individual was 95.2%.
- The non-significant excess of males in our patient population confirms similar finding by 3 other investigators.
- In HLA and disease association studies, clinical diagnoses should be confirmed by histological studies, whenever possible.

Acknowledgements

We wish to thank the staff of the Department of Immunohaematology of the Leyden University Hospital for their help with HLA typings, Mrs. D. de Wolff-Rouendaal, Department of Pathology of the Leyden University Eye Clinic and Dr. M. Gorsira, Department of Pathology of the Diaconessenhuis for the histological examinations.

References

Blagojevic M., Szanojevic-Paovic A., Susakovic N. and Orlic M. 1980. HLA antigens and keratoconus. The Cornea in Health and Disease VI the Congress of European Society of Opthalmol). The Royal Soc. of Medicine and Acc. Press London No. 40: 937-940.

D'Amaro J., Van Rood J.J., Rimm A.A. and Bortin M.M. (1983) HLA associations in Italian and non-Italian Caucasoid aplastic anaemia patients. Tissue Antigens 21: 184-191.

Damgaard-Jensen L., Ehlers N & Kissmeyer Nielsen F. (1979) HLA types in corneal diseases. Acta Ophthal. 57: 982-985.

Edwards J.H. (1974) HLA and disease. The detection of associations. J. of Immunogenet. 1: 249.

Fasset A.R., Richman A.V., Frias J.L. (1977). HLA antigens and keratoconus. Ann. of Ophthalmol. 9: 767-768.
Grayson M. (1979) Degenerations, dystrophies and edema of the cornea. In Duane TD (ed) Clinical Ophthalmology Harper and Row Publishers, Hagerstown, Cambridge 4, 6: 20-21.
Karantinos D., Louletzoglon M., Stavropoulon K., Apostolopoulos M., Renieri N. and Theodossiadis G. Histocompatibility Antigens (HLA) in keratoconus (1980). The Cornea in Health and Disease (VIIth Congress of European Society of Ophthalmol.) The Royal Soc. of Medicine and Ac. Press. London 40: 933-936.
Klouda P.T., Syrbopoulos E.K., Entwhistle C.C., Coffin R.B., Easty P.L. and Brandley B.A. (1983) HLA and keratoconus. Tissue Antigens 21: 397-399.
Nijenhuis L.E. (1961) Blood group frequencies in The Netherlands, Curacao, Suriname and New Guinea. A study in population genetics. Thesis, University Amsterdam.
Vannas S., Vannas A. and Tiilikainen A. (1977). Corneal transplantation reaction in avascular keratoconus patients due to HLA-associated immune aberation against infection. Invest. Ophthalmol. Visual Sci. 644-646.
Völker-Dieben H.J., D'Amaro J., de Lange P. and Wolff-Rouendaal D. (1983). HLA and ABO antigens in malignant choroidal melanonia. Clin. exp. Immunol 53: 581-588.
Wachtmeister L., Ingemansson S., and Möller E. Atopy and HLA antigens in patients with keratoconus. Acta Ophthalmol. 60: 113-122.

CHAPTER 14

HLA and ABO antigens in patients with Fuchs' endothelial dystrophy*

Summary

Twenty-three patients with Fuchs' dystrophy and 200 controls were studied for the distribution of HLA-A, -B and -C antigens. HLA-A3, -B18, -B27 and -Cw2 were found to be significantly more frequent before correction for the 30 antigens studied.

Introduction

Fuchs' dystrophy, also called primairy endothelial decompensation of the cornea, is a condition which may be hereditary and is usually dominantly transmitted (Krachmer et al. 1978). The endothelial cells demonstrate functional regression with age, mostly in female patients in the fifth or six decade of life (Doggart 1957). Because of the frequently observed familial character of the disease, we decided to investigate if there were any significant associations between the disease and HLA, the most polymorphic genetic system known in man. Damgaard-Jensen et al. (1979) reported a borderline (uncorrected) significantly elevated frequency for HLA-B12 in 23 patients with Fuchs' dystrophy. We also examined the distribution of ABO antigens since a significant difference in the O and non-O blood group had been observed in patients with malignant choroidal melanoma (chapter 15).

Material and methods

Twenty-three Dutch patients (12 male and 11 female) and 200 healthy unrelated Dutch controls of Caucasoid origin were the subject of this study. The patients were tissue typed prior to a penetrating keratoplasty. The corneal buttons excised at the time of transplantation were examined histologically. The clinical diagnosis was confirmed in all cases (Wolff-Rouendaal et al. 1981). The ages of the patients ranged from 52 to 88 years, average 63.0 years.

* *For colour plates, see pp. 72ff.*

Typing for 8 HLA-A, 16 HLA-B and 6 HLA-C antigens was performed by using a standard microlymphocytotoxicity assay (Van Rood 1979). All HLA typings of the patients and the controls were performed in the National Reference Centre in Leyden (Department of Immunohaematology, University Hospital) with a serum set which recognizes all official HLA and Workshop A, B and C specificities. The ABO blood groups of the 23 patients were determined in the bloodbank of the University Hospital.

The HLA phenotypes of the 23 patients with Fuchs' dystrophy were analysed for possible associations with the HLA-A, -B and -C locus antigens. The HLA frequencies of the patient group were compared to those of a control group of 200 healthy unrelated Dutch Caucaso individuals typed in the same laboratory by the same technicians. Haldane's (1955) modifications of Woolfs method (1955) was used to estimate the significance of the

Table 1. Woolf-Haldane analysis of the HLA antigen frequencies in 23 patients with Fuchs's dystrophy

Antigen	Patients pos.	neg.	Controls pos.	neg.	Relative risk	Chi. square	p value
A1	7	16	68	132	0.879	0.080	0.769
A2	12	11	105	95	0.984	0.001	0.921
A3	11	12	51	149	2.671	5.184	0.022*
A9	2	21	39	161	0.475	1.349	0.244
A10	2	21	7	193	3.000	2.371	0.120
A11	3	20	25	175	1.175	0.076	0.774
A28	4	19	17	183	2.420	2.511	0.109
Aw19	3	20	46	154	0.567	0.988	0.322
B5	1	22	24	176	0.480	0.913	0.342
B7	7	16	51	149	1.320	0.367	0.552
B8	3	20	45	155	0.583	0.891	0.348
B12	7	16	60	140	1.056	0.014	0.872
B13	0	23	6	194	0.637	0.171	0.682
B14	1	22	8	192	1.510	0.257	0.618
B15	4	19	31	169	1.242	0.163	0.688
Bw16	1	22	14	186	0.857	0.038	0.825
B17	2	21	20	180	1.024	0.001	0.922
B18	5	18	15	185	3.558	5.609	0.017*
Bw21	1	22	3	197	3.762	2.198	0.134
Bw22	0	23	9	191	0.429	0.625	0.435
B27	5	18	15	185	3.558	5.609	0.017*
Bw35	3	20	35	165	0.796	0.157	0.694
B37	2	21	7	193	3.000	2.371	0.120
B40	2	21	25	175	0.800	0.117	0.730
Cw1	1	22	7	193	1.720	0.437	0.516
Cw2	6	17	17	182	3.873	7.068	0.008*
Cw3	3	20	62	137	0.376	2.989	0.080
Cw4	3	20	39	159	0.689	0.421	0.524
Cw5	1	18	30	165	0.440	1.141	0.285
Cw6	4	9	26	154	2.762	3.004	0.079

* Significant p values before correction for the 30 antigens studied.

different antigen frequencies in these patients and controls. P values were corrected, whenever appropriate, for a total of 30 HLA antigens using the procedure suggested by Edwards (1974).

For all antigens with no occurrence in a patient population, the probability of their occurrence was calculated as follows. If the antigen frequency in the control group is PF, then the random chance of its occurrence in the patient population is PF and the chance of its non-occurrence is 1-PF. It then follows that the probability of at least one occurrence of the antigen in N patients is $1-(1-PF)^N$.

Results

HLA associations

In 23 patients with Fuchs' dystrophy HLA-A3, B18, B27 and CW2 were significantly elevated but not after correction (see table 1).

ABO blood groups

The distribution of the ABO blood groups was not significantly different in the 12 male and 11 female patients with Fuchs' dystrophy (table 2). In addition, the ABO blood group distribution in the total patient group was not significantly different from that in the Dutch control population (Nijenhuis, 1961).

Sex and age distributions

There was no significant difference in the numbers of males and females in the patient population. A slight but not significant difference in age was observed in the group of male patients versus female patients. The ages of the male patients ranged from 37 to 82, average 57.5 years, while the ages of the female patients ranged from 60 to 88, average 73.3 years.

Table 2. ABO blood groups in 23 patients with Fuchs' dystrophy

		Blood group			
	N	O	A	B	AB
Male	12	4	7	1	0
Female	11	5	6	0	0
Total	23	9	13	1	0

Discussion

The lack of significant HLA antigen associations after correction for the number of antigens tested in patients with Fuchs' dystrophy agrees with the primary conclusion of Damgaard Jensen et al. (1979) namely, that there were no significant associations. Their observation of a significant HLA-B12 antigen frequency (uncorrected) was not confirmed by us.

There were no significant differences in the distributions of the ABO antigens in the males and females nor in the combined patients as compared to the control Dutch population.

Finally, in contrast to the report by Doggart (1957), there was no excess of females in our patient population. Furthermore the age distribution of the females were higher than those of the males but not significantly.

Conclusions

Significantly elevated HLA-A3, -B18, -B27 and -Cw2 antigen frequencies, before correction, were observed in 23 patients with Fuchs' dystrophy. After correction for the total of 30 comparisons, the number of HLA-A, -B and -C antigens studied, the antigen frequency deviations were no longer significant.

Acknowledgements

We wish to thank the staff of the Department of Immunohaematology of the Leyden University Hospital for their help with HLA typings, Mrs. D. de Wolff-Rouendaal, Department of Pathology of the Leyden University Eye Clinic, Dr. M. Gorsira, Department of Pathology of the Diaconessenhuis for the histological examinations.

References

Damgaard-Jensen L., Ehlers N and Kissmeyer Nielsen F. (1979) HLA types in corneal diseases. Acta Ophthal. 57: 982-985.

Doggart J.H. (1957) Fuchs' epithelial dystrophy of the cornea. Brit J. ophthal. 41: 533-540.

Edwards J.H. (1974) HLA and disease. The detection of associations. J. Immunogenet. 1: 249.

Haldane J.B.S. (1955) The estimation and significance of the logarithm of ratio of frequencies. Am. Hum. Genet. 20: 30.

Krachmer J.H., Purcell Jr. J.J., Young C.W. and Buchner K.D. (1978) Corneal endothelial dystrophy. Arch. ophthalmol 96: 2036-2039.

Nijenhuis L.E. (1961) Blood group frequencies in the Netherlands, Curacao, Suriname and New Guinea. A study in population genetics. Thesis, University Amsterdam.

Van Rood J.J. (1979) Microlymphocytotoxicity method. In: NIAID Manual of tissue typing techniques (Ed: J. Ray) National Institute of Health (NIH) (80-545) Maryland, U.S.A.: p. 104.

Wolff-Rouendaal de D., Völker-Dieben H.J. and Kok-Van Alphen C.C. (1981). The histology of iatrogenic keratitis bullosa. Doc. Ophthalmol 50: 357-364.

Woolf B. (1955) On estimating the relation between bloodgroups and disease. Ann. Hum. Genet. 19: 251.

CHAPTER 15

HLA and ABO antigens in patients with malignant choroidal melanoma*

Summary

Comparisons of the HLA antigen frequencies in normal controls and in different subsets of patients with malignant choroidal melanoma, partitioned on the basis of histological tumour cell types and inclusion of the splits of all of the HLA-A and -B locus antigens, revealed significant heterogeneity only in HLA-B (p=0.043) in the 'pure spindle' cell type choroidal melanomas. In the 'not pure spindle' cell type choroidal melanomas, borderline heterogenity in HLA-B (p=0.064) was observed. A comparison of the HLA antigen frequencies in the 'pure' and 'not pure spindle' cell choroidal melanoma patients revealed only one antigen with a significant difference before correction, namely B27. A significant difference in ABO bloodgroup distributions, divided into O and non-O, in the two tumour classes was observed (Exact p(1)=0.0036).

Introduction

There have been numerous studies on HLA antigen associations in patients with different ophthalmic disorders - for a review see Bertrams et al. (1978). An overview of HLA antigen association studies in patients with a malignant choroidal melanoma and their results are set out in table 1. In the above reports, the splits of the HLA-A locus antigens were partially analyzed but the splits of the HLA-B locus antigens were not analyzed. In only one study were the patients grouped into different subsets on the basis of histological cell types (Ignatov et al. 1977).

Paul et al. (1962) described a striking difference in clinical course in relation to different tumour cell types. The 15 year mortality rates were 19%

Table 1. Overview of HLA antigen association studies in patients with malignant choroidal melanoma

Author	Number of patients	Antigens
Ignatov et al. (1977)	47	A3(ns A29(ns)
Bertrams et al. (1978)	81	Aw32
Dieckhues et al. (1979)	5	–

* *For colour plates, see pp. 72ff.*

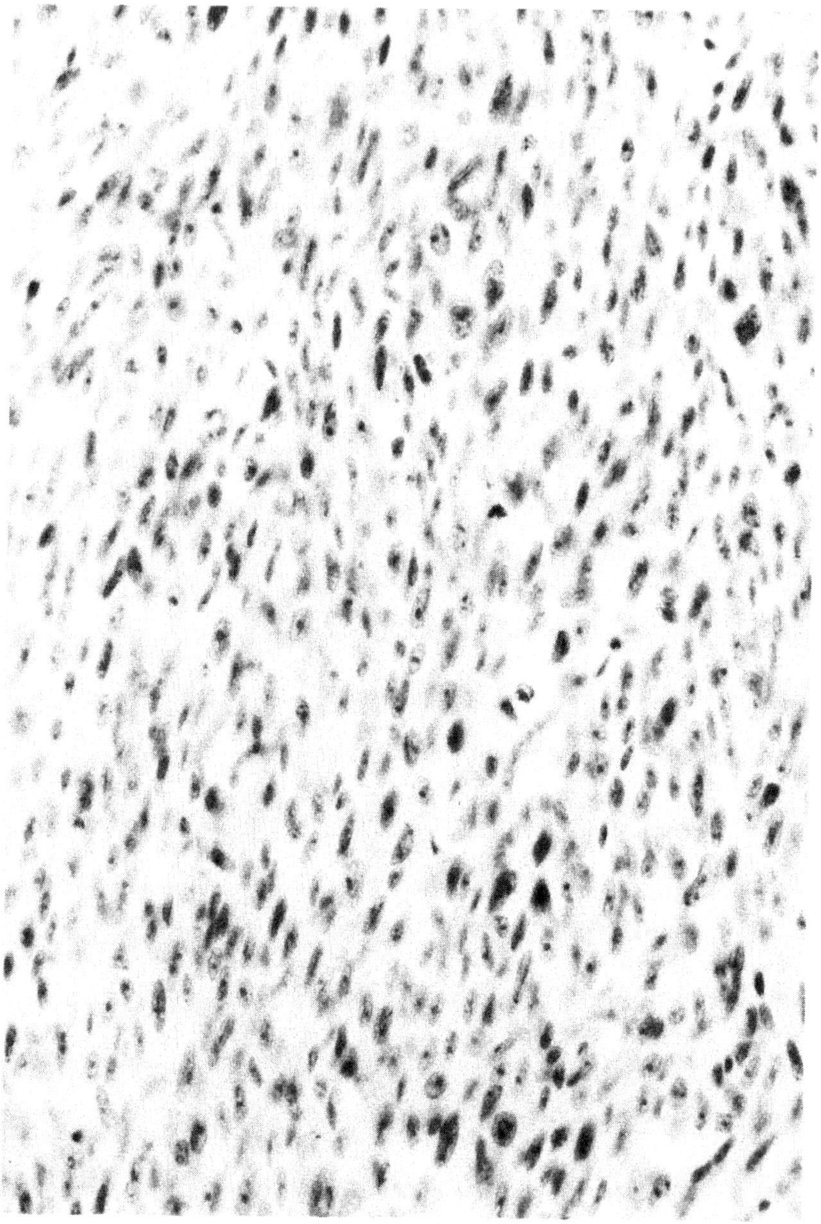

Figure 1. Melanoma chorioidea spindle cell type closely packed cells with oval nuclei and distinct nucleolus (magnification x 400).

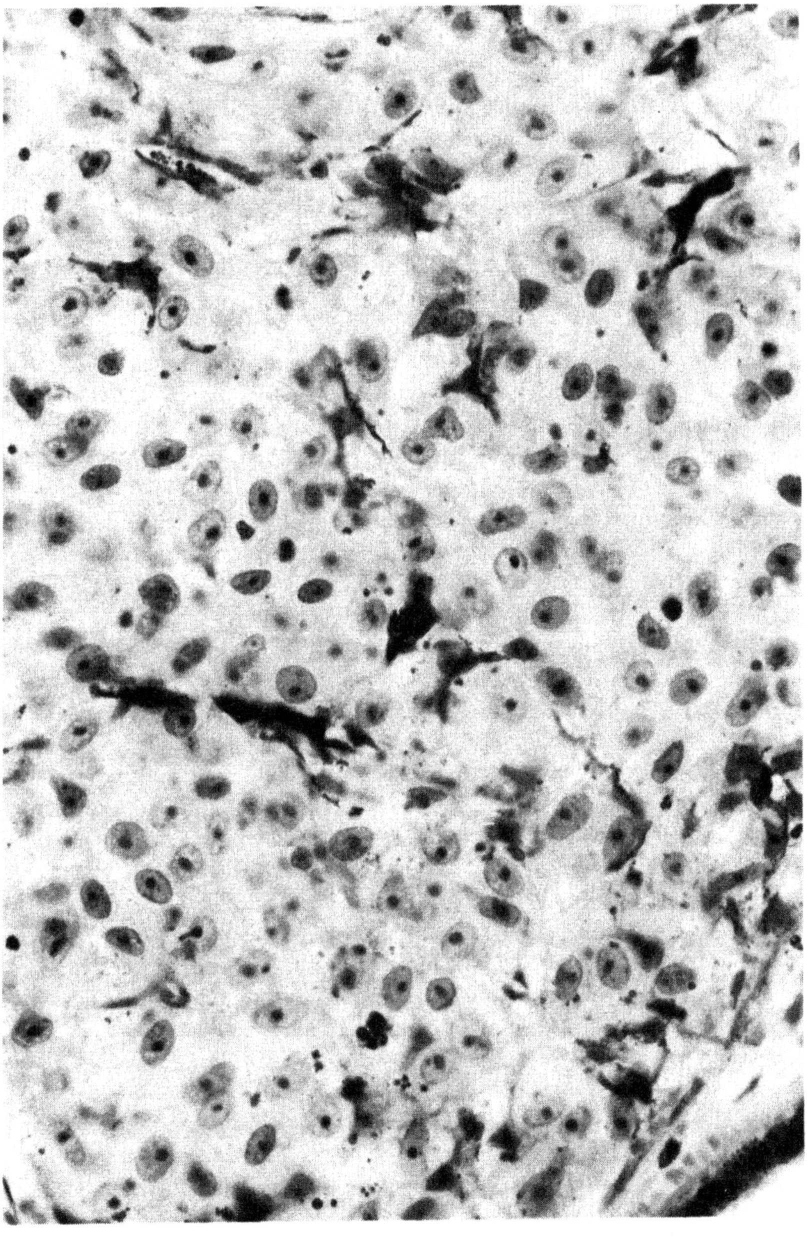

Figure 2. Melanoma chorioidea epitheloid cell type closely packed cells with abundant cytoplasm, round or oval nuclei and very large nucleotus (magnification x 400).

and 25% for the spindle A and B cell types respectively ('pure spindle cell type', fig. 1) compared to 59% and 72% in the mixed and epitheloid cell tumours respectively ('not pure spindle cell type', fig. 2).

There are indications that patients with malignant melanoma react against their tumours and that this reaction may have an immunological basis (Lewis 1972, Mavligit et al. (1974). Immune responsiveness is under control by genes in the Major Histocompatibility Complex (McDevitt 1969). For that reason, we analyzed the HLA antigen frequencies in patients with 'pure spindle cell' tumours and 'not pure spindle cell' type tumours separately, since there are marked differences in the 15 year mortality rates of patients with those two tumour types.

We included all of the 'splits' of the HLA antigens in our analyses because they had not been studied previously. The fact that this study was retrospective and the more urgent priorities in the typing laboratory prevented us from obtaining DR typings for the melanoma patients.

Joycey et al. (1973) have suggested that blood group O individuals may be relatively immuno-incompetent. Therefore, we decided to extend our study to include the ABO antigens to see if we could confirm those hypotheses.

Material and methods

Sixty-nine Dutch patients and 1018 healthy Dutch controls of Caucasoid origin were the subjects of this study. Typing for 14 HLA-A, 24 HLA-B and 6 HLA-C antigens was performed by using a standard micro lymphocytotoxicity assay (Van Rood 1979). All HLA typings of the patients and the controls were performed in the National Reference Center in Leyden (Department of Immunohaematology, University Hospital) with the Eurotransplant serum set which recognizes all official HLA and Workshop A and B specificities. The ABO blood groups of 68 patients were determined in the blood bank of the University Hospital. The HLA phenotypes of the 69 patients with malignant choroidal melanoma were analyzed for possible associations with the HLA-A, -B and -C antigens. The HLA frequencies of the patient group were compared to those of a control group of 1018 normal Dutch individuals typed in the same laboratory by the same technicians. The Woolf-Haldane (Woolf, Haldane 1955) analysis was used to estimate the significance of the different antigen frequencies in these patients and controls. P values were corrected, whenever appropriate, for a total of 44 HLA antigens using the procedure suggested by Edwards (1974).

Multiplex testing for heterogenity in the frequencies of all antigens in a single locus was performed by summing the chi squares, which is itself a chi square with degrees of freedom equal to the number of antigens in the locus (Svejgaard et al. 1974). For all antigens with no occurrence in a patient population, the probability of occurrence was calculated as follows. If the antigen frequency in the control group is PF, then the random chance of its occurrence in the patient population is PF and the chance of its non-occurrence is 1-PF. It then follows that probability of at least one occurrence of the antigen in N patients is $1-(1-PF)^N$.

In all 69 patients, 34 male patients and 35 females, the affected eye was enucleated. None of the patients had a bilateral choroidal melanoma. The diagnosis of malignant choroidal melanoma was based on the histologic examination of the tissue, classified according to Callendar et al. (1942), performed by the Department of Pathology. None of the patients had been treated with light or laser coagulation, nor had they received systemic immunosuppressive therapy before enucleation of the bulbus. The ages of the patients ranged from 9 to 83 years, average 57.6 years.

Results

HLA associations

In 69 patients with malignant choroidal melanoma, only HLA-Bw49 was elevated and significantly different before correction (Relative Risk (R.R.) = 5.769, X^2=6.244, p=0.012). These 69 patients were divided into two classes according to the histological cell types of their tumours. 35 Tumours consisted of Spindle cells only (pure spindle cell tumour) (fig. 1), no epitheloid cells were found. The remaining 34 tumours contained epitheloid cells only in 8 cases and 26 tumours consisted of both epitheloid and spindle cells. These 34 tumours will be described as 'not pure spindle cell tumours' (fig. 2).

In the 'pure spindle' group, multiplex testing revealed significant heterogenity only in HLA-B (X^2=37.309, d.f.=24, p=0.043). The greatest contributions to the heterogenity were made by Bw51 (R.R.=3.388), Bw63 (R.R.=9.802) and Bw49 (R.R.=6.773). In the HLA-A locus only Aw30 was significantly elevated (R.R.=3.739). None of these associations remained significant after correction for the total of 44 comparisons. There were 11 antigens which were never positive in those patients. It is interesting to note that the random chance of observing one positive reaction in that patient population was 80% or more for Aw31 (91,7%) and B27 (92,5%) (see Table 2).

In the 'not pure spindle' group, multiplex testing revealed no significant heterogenity in HLA-A (p=0.447) and borderline heterogenity in HLA-B (p=0.064). Bw38 (R.R.=4.949) was elevated, but not significantly after correction for the 44 comparisons. There were 12 antigens which were never positive in these patients. Only three of them had a random chance greater than 80% of being detected in that patient population A29 (83,9%), Aw30 (84,9%) and Bw57 (93,8%) (see Table 2).

A comparison of the HLA antigen frequencies in the 'pure' and 'not pure

Table 2. Distribution of HLA antigens in patients with 'pure spindle cell' and 'non pure spindle cell' choroidal melanoma and in healthy Dutch Caucasoid controls

Antigen	Pure Spindle Pos	Neg	Non-pure Spindle Pos	Neg	Controls Pos	Neg
A1	13	21	14	20	318	700
A2	17	18	14	20	535	483
A3	7	28	10	24	296	722
Aw23	0	32	0	33	24	989
Aw24	5	27	4	29	173	835
A25	1	34	2	32	17	1001
A26	1	34	2	32	43	975
A11	4	31	4	30	112	905
A28	6	29	5	29	97	913
A29	1	34	0	34	46	972
Aw30	4	31	0	34	37	981
Aw31	0	35	2	32	70	948
Aw32	2	33	2	32	55	962
Aw33	0	35	0	34	15	1002
Bw51	5	15	1	21	96	921
Bw52	0	20	0	22	6	1007
B7	9	26	8	26	282	736
B8	12	23	10	24	244	774
Bw44	7	28	4	30	246	771
Bw45	0	35	0	34	16	1002
B13	1	34	1	33	44	974
B14	1	34	2	32	30	987
Bw63	1	34	0	34	4	1014
Bw62	4	31	6	28	170	845
Bw38	0	35	4	30	29	989
Bw39	2	33	2	32	42	976
Bw57	1	10	0	10	52	959
Bw58	0	11	0	10	12	997
B18	2	33	1	33	73	945
Bw49	1	34	1	33	6	1012
Bw50	0	35	0	34	11	1004
Bw55	2	18	1	21	40	978
Bw56	0	20	0	22	8	1008
B27	0	35	5	29	69	949
Bw35	8	27	5	29	175	843
B37	0	35	3	31	45	972
Bw61	1	33	0	32	30	978
Bw60	5	29	3	29	157	861
Cw1	1	32	1	33	56	962
Cw2	3	32	4	29	94	916
Cw3	10	25	9	24	351	662
Cw4	9	26	6	28	215	797
Cw5	2	28	2	28	106	901
Cw6	3	12	4	13	131	733

spindle cell' choroidal melanoma patients revealed only one antigen with a significant difference before correction, namely B27 (exact $p(2) = 0.05$). Since that antigen was present in only one of those patient groups, we determined the random chance of its occurrence in the other group. The results yielded a value of 99.6 percent.

ABO Blood groups

The distribution of the ABO blood groups was not significantly different in the 34 male and 35 female patients with malignant choroidal melanoma. In addition, the ABO blood group distribution in the total patient group was not significantly different from that in the Dutch control population.

Table 3. ABO Bloodgroups in 2 Choroidal Melanoma histological Cell Types

	BLOOD GROUP				
Tumor Cell Type	A	B	AB	O*	Non-O*
Pure Spindle (n=35)	17	5	2	11	24
Non-pure Spindle (n=33)	8	3	0	22	11

$X^2 = 9.76$, $p(2) = 0.021$
* O vs Non-O: Exact $p(1) = 0.0036$

Table 3 shows the relation between ABO blood groups and the histological types of the tumour cells. The distribution of the blood groups is only slightly significantly different from the expectations ($p=0.021$). However, when the blood groups are divided into O and non-O classes in an attempt to confirm Joycey's hypothesis, a highly significant difference in their distribution in the two tumour classes is observed (exact $p(1) = 0.0036$). There is a relative excess of the non-O in the 'pure spindle' group and a relative excess of O in the 'not pure spindle' group.

Sex distribution

There are relatively more pure spindle cell cases in female patients, but the difference is not significant.

Discussion

HLA antigens

The lack of significantly increased HLA antigen associations in patients with malignant choroidal melanoma in our study does not agree with the results of Ignatov et al. (1977) who studied 47 patients, and Bertrams et al. (1978) who studied 81 patients.

Ignatov et al. (1977) reported increased frequencies of HLA-A3 and HLA-A29 and decreased frequencies of HLA-A25 and HLA-Bw16 in 47 patients with choroidal melanoma. In addition, there is some uncertainty about his patient and control populations. He refers only to 'patients' and to 'healthy donors' from Odessa. Even if the subjects were all Caucasoids, that would not exclude population heterogeneity. Furthermore, the diagnosis of malignant choroidal melanoma was based on histological examination in only 25 of his 47 patients. The diseased eyes of the remaining 22 patients were not enucleated. Diagnosis of these patients was based only on ophthalmological examination and clinical picture.

Bertrams et al. (1978) reported an increased frequency of HLA-Aw32 (p=0.001) in 81 patients with choroidal melanoma as compared to 1000 normal controls. Patients and controls were all referred to as Caucasoids. After correction for the total number of antigens studied, this p value was still significant (p=0.026). The diagnosis of malignant choroidal melanoma was based on microscopic examination of tissue from enucleated eyes in all 81 cases. No analyses were performed on patients with different histological cell types.

In our own material, we have made a subdivision of the malignant choroidal melanoma cases according to their histological diagnosis. Our results revealed an absence of B27 in the 'pure spindle' subset. Our studies of the HLA-A and -B low antigenic splits revealed no significant heterogenety, after correction, neither between the 2 patient subsets, nor between those groups and the healthy controls.

Our analysis of patients subsets, classified on the basis of histological tumour cell types and the inclusion of antigenic splits may explain the differences between previous reports and our results.

ABO blood groups

Lamm et al. (1974) reported a comparison of the results of HLA and ABO typing in 212 malignant melanoma patients and those obtained from 562 healthy controls. The distribution of the ABO antigens in the malignant melanoma patients as a whole and in the subgroups divided according to sex and prognosis for survival, showed no significant deviation from the distribution in 562 controls. No subdivision according to the cell type was made.

In our study of 69 patients with malignant choroidal melanoma, we confirmed the results of Lamm. No significant deviation in the ABO blood group distribution was found when the patients, irrespective of histologic tumour cell type, were compared to the Dutch control population. However, when the malignant choroidal melanoma patients are subdivided according to the histological types of their tumours, a slightly significant difference from the expectations is observed (Table 3, p=0.021) and a highly significant difference is observed when the blood groups are partitioned into O and non-O classes (exact p(1) = 0.0036).

Lewis (1972) and Mavligit et al. (1974) have suggested that there is an immunological basis for the reaction of melanoma patients against their tumours. Furthermore, blood group O individuals may be relatively immuno-incompetent(Joycey 1973). Our finding of a relative excess of blood group O patients with 'not pure spindle' choroidal melanoma is consistent with those 2 hypothesis since that tumor type is more malignant than the 'pure spindle' type.

Clinical considerations

In 1978, Zimmerman et al. reported that enucleation may have an adverse effect with respect to the development of metastatic disease in patients with choroidal melanoma. Their observations have re-stimulated the discussion as to whether or not to enucleate or only to observe small choroidal melanomas (for review see Manschot and Van Peperzeel (1980).

The four most important factors concerning the prognosis of malignant melanoma of the choroid are:cell type; tumour size; degree of mitotic activity and scleral extension. Except for the tumour size, the other three variables are established only by histological examination of the enucleated eye. Unfortunately for the clinician, there is no correlation between tumour size and cell type (Flocks et al. 1955, Davidorf and Lang 1974 and Jensen 1970). Hagler et al. (1977) were unable to demonstrate any significant correlation between ^{32}P test results and histological cell types, although it was to be expected that more malignant tumours would have a higher metabolic rate and thus a higher ^{32}P uptake.

Conclusions

- HLA-A, -B and -C typing of 69 patients with malignant choroidal melanoma revealed a significantly elevated frequency of Bw49 before correction for the total of 44 antigens studied.
- Malignant choroidal melanoma of the '*not* pure spindle cell type' was associated with a significantly elevated frequency of Bw38 before correction.
- Comparison of the HLA antigen frequencies in the 'pure' and 'not pure spindle cell' choroidal melanoma patients revealed only one antigen with a significant difference before correction: B27 was observed only in the 'not pure spindle cell type'.
- When the blood groups are partitioned into O and not-O classes, a highly significant difference in their distribution in the two tumour classes was observed. Blood group O was increased in the more malignant 'not pure spindle cell type' and not-O in the less malignant 'pure spindle cell type'.

- No significant differential sex distribution was observed in the 69 patients with malignant choroidal melanoma as a whole nor in two patient subgroups, partitioned according to histological tumour cell types.
- Cell type is recognized as the most important prognostic factor for malignant melanoma of the choroid. Information on the ABO blood groups from such patients may be predictive of the histological cell types of the tumours and help clinicians in their decision as to whether or not to enucleate the eye. The prognostic value of HLA still remains to be determined. Our admittedly tentative findings should be examined for eventual confirmation in other centers.

Acknowledgements

We wish to acknowledge the assistence of the Department of Medical Statistics of the Leyden University, especially Dr. J. Hermans.

References

Bertrams J., Spitznas M. and Rommelfanger M. (1978) Missing evidence for HLA antigen association with Eales' disease, chorioretinitis, central serous retinopathy and malignant choroidal melanoma. Invest. Ophthalmol. 17: 9, 918-920.

Callendar G.R, Wilder H.C, Esh J.E. (1942) Five hundred melanomas of the choroid and ciliary body followed five years or longer. American Journal Ophthal. 25: 962-967.

Davidorf F.H, Lang J.R. (1974) Small malignant melanomas of the choroid. Am. J. Ophthalmol. 78: 788-793.

Dieckhues B., Jümann G., Küchle H.J., Püttmann T. (1979) HLA Antigene bei Augenerkrankungen. Klin. Mbl. Augenheilk. 175: 681-685.

Edwards J.H. (1974) HL-A and disease. The detection of associations. J. of Immunogenetics 1: 249.

Flocks M., Gerende J.H., Zimmerman L.E. (1955) The size and shape of the choroid and ciliary body in relation to the prognosis and histologic characteristics. Trans. Am. Acad. Ophthalmol. Otolaryngol. 59: 740-758.

Hagler W.S., Jarret W.H. and Killian J.H. (1977) The use of the 32P test in the management of malignant melanoma of the choroid. Tr. Am. Acad. Ophthalmol. and Otolaryngol. 83: 49-60.

Haldane J.B.S. (1955) The estimation and significance of the logarithm of ratio of frequencies. Ann. Hum. Genet. 20: 30.

Ignatov R.K., Terentyevra L.L., Shulgina N.S. (1977) A study of antigen distribution of HLA system in melanoma of the uvea (Russian). Onkologiceskij Zurnal, 14: 289.

Jensen O.A. (1970) Malignant melanomas of the human uvea. Recent follow-up of cases in Denmark 1943-1952. Acta Ophthalmol. 48: 1113-1128.

Joycey V.C., Roger J.H., Evans D.B., Hebertson B.M. (1973) Kidney graft survival and matching for HLA and ABO antigens. Nature 246: 163.

Lamm L.U., Kissmeyer-Nielsen F., Kjerbye K.E., Mogensen B. and Petersen N.C. (1974) HLA and ABO antigens and malignant melanoma. Cancer 33: 1458-1461.

Lewis M.G. (1972) Immunology of human malignant melanoma. In: Immunological Aspects of neoplasia II. Series Haematologica V 5: p. 44-65, Munksgaard, Copenhagen.

Manschot W.A. and Van Peperzeel A. (1980) Choroidal melanoma, Enucleation or observation? A new approach. Arch Ophthalmol. 98: 71-77.

Mavligit G., Guttermann J.U., Mc Bride C. and Hersh E.M. (1974) Tumor directed immune reactivity and immuno therapy in malignant melanoma. Current status. Immunology of Cancer. Prog. Exp. Tumor Res. 19: 222-252.

McDevitt H.O and Chinnitz A. (1969) Genetic control of the antibody response: relationship between immune response and Histocompatibility (H-2) type. Science 163: 1207-1208.

Paul E.V., Parnell B.L. and Fraher M. (1962) 'Prognosis of malignant melanomas of the choroid and ciliary body'. Int. Ophthalmological Clinics 2: 387.

Van Rood J.J. (1979) Microlymphocytotoxicity method. In: NIAID Manual of tissue typing techniques (Ed: J. Ray) National Institute of Health (NIH) (80-545) Maryland, U.S.A.: p. 104.

Svejgaard A. et al. (1974) HL-A antigens and disease. Statistical and genetical considerations. Tissue Antigens 4: 95-105.

Woolf B. (1955) On estimating the relation between blood groups and disease. Ann. Hum. Genet. 19: 251,

Zimmerman L.E., McLean J.W., Foster W.D. (1978) Does enucleation of the eye containing a malignant melanoma prevent or accelerate the dissemination of tumor cells? Br. J. Ophthalmol. 62: 420-425.

CHAPTER 16

Summary and general discussion*

The objective of this thesis was to study factors influencing corneal graft survival. These factors can be classified as non-immunological or immunological.

The main non-immunological factor which has increased graft survival since 1939 is the improvement in surgical techniques following the introduction of the operation microscope. A linear relation between the improved surgical skill and the number of less favourable cases which could be operated was observed in many corneal transplantation centers. Patients with highly vascularized corneas and previous corneal graft failures were no longer excluded from corneal transplantation. At the present time, corneal graft rejection due to immunological factors is the ultimate determinant of corneal graft survival.

Of the immunological factors which may influence corneal graft survival, we have studied the effect of the major histocompatibility complex (MHC) and theABO blood group system. The human MHC (HLA) is a genetic system that contains information for polymorphic cell membrane determinants. HLA antigenic incompatibilities provoke strong immunological reactions in tissue transplantation. Furthermore, genes within the HLA-system influence the individual degree of susceptibility to diseases implicating the immune system.

The results of our studies will be summarized and discussed following the outline as described in the introduction (chapter 1).

Section I

The ultimate limitation for all organ or tissue transplantations is the availability of donor material. Corneas from living donors i.e. corneas obtained from eyes enucleated because of a malignant choroidal melanoma (MCM) were the key to the start of corneal transplantation in The Netherlands in 1939 and to the start of prospectively HLA-A and -B matched corneal transplants in 1976. The suitability of donor corneas obtained from eyes enucleated because of MCM was evaluated in a long term follow-up

* *For colour plates, see pp. 72ff.*

study (chapter 3) and in a comparative study of corneas from donors deceased because of systemic malignancies (chapter 4).

The long term follow-up study revealed no evidence for the transmission of tumour cells by corneal transplantation. A negative effect on the life expectancies of the recipients of this donor material could not be established (chapter 3). Nevertheless, the use of such corneal grafts is not advised, since a lower graft survival of the donor corneas obtained from eyes enucleated because of MCM was observed when compared to the graft survival of corneas obtained from donors with systemic malignancies. The only significant difference in causes of graft failure in the two study groups was an elevated number of irreversible rejections in the grafts obtained from eyes enucleated because of MCM (chapter 4).

Section II

The effect of numerous non-HLA factors on graft survival were evaluated (chapter 5).

Previous graft failure, high degree of corneal vascularization and large corneal graft diameters are associated with relatively short graft survival times as compared to transplantations performed in their absence.

Blood group O recipients of corneas from blood group A donors had a better graft survival than other ABO donor-recipient combinations.

The effect of donor-recipient sex combinations was significant only when corneas from female donors were used. Corneal graft survival was significantly better in female recipients of such corneas than in male recipients.

Previous pregnancies, blood transfusions, donor age and cause of death of the donor, time interval between donor death and transplantation and storage methods (chapter 5).

Blood group O recipients of corneas from blood group A donors had a better graft survival than other ABO donor-recipient combinations.

The effect of donor-recipient sex combinations was significant only when corneas from female donors were used. Corneal graft survival was significantly better in female recipients of such corneas than in male recipients.

Previous pregnancies, blood transfusions, donor age and cause of death of the donor, time interval between donor death and transplantation and storage methods did not influence the survival of corneal grafts (chapter 5).

These results have relevance for the study of the effect of prospective HLA-A and -B matching on corneal graft survival (chapter 6). Prospective HLA-A and -B matching results in a significantly improved graft survival rate in patients with vascularized corneas and in patients who have rejected previous grafts.

The beneficial effect of HLA-DR matching on kidney graft survival prompted us to study this effect on corneal graft survival (chapter 7). HLA-DR matching did not significantly influence corneal graft survival. However, there is a highly significant difference in the survival of small versus large grafts. That difference is seen predominantly in vascularized recipient corneas, but smaller grafts do better, although not significantly, than larger grafts in non vascularized corneas (chapter 7). These observations are consistent with the fact that HLA-DR antigens are found only in the perifery of the cornea.

The studies reported in chapter 5, 6 and 7 were performed on the complete data. The following 3 chapters report the results of studies performed in specific subsets of these patients.

In chapter 8 the surgical and postoperative problems in keratoplasties in children are described. Corneal graft survival in children between the ages of 3 and 15 years is comparable to that in adults. There were no significant differences in the survival of corneas from young or adult donors in pediatric or adult recipients. Corneal graft rejections were not observed in the HLA-A and -B matched donor-recipient combinations. However, high levels of complications are observed in pediatric recipients i.e. anterior displacement of the irisdiaphragma and lens during the operative procedure and frequent infections in the post-operative period. On the other hand, lower degrees of astigmatism were seen in the pediatric patients than is normally seen in adult patients.

Endothelial decompensation is observed as a primary corneal disease (or Fuchs' dystrophy) and as a secondary corneal disease after the performance of anterior segment surgery. Cataract extraction, whether or not in combination with intraocular lens insertion, may lead to secondary endothelial decompensation (or bullous keratoplasty). The most effective treatment for these diseases is corneal transplantation. Chapter 9 describes the results of corneal transplantation for primary and secondary endothelial decompensation and of the influence of an intraocular lens on corneal graft survival. There were no significant differences in the survival of corneal grafts in patients with secondary endothelial decompensation as compared to their survival in the rest of the patients nor in patients with primary (P.E.D.) versus secondary endothelial decompensation (S.E.D.). However, the graft survival in patients with S.E.D. was lower than that in the non-decompensated and the P.E.D. patients. In S.E.D. patients, the presence of an implant lens has an adverse effect on the survival of corneal grafts. Nevertheless, it is not advised to remove every implant lens at the time of graft surgery because the inevitable surgical trauma may cause cystoid macular edema and a reduction in visual acuity.

Recurrent herpes simplex virus (HSV) keratitis results in scar formation and blood vessel ingrowth in the cornea. The majority of the HSV keratitis patients for whom corneal transplantation is indicated show severely vascularized corneas. We presumed that these patients would benefit from HLA-A and -B matched grafts. Chapter 10 shows that the fate of corneal transplants performed because of herpetic keratitis is inversely proportional to the degree of recipient corneal vascularisation. In the same patient group, HLA-A and -B matched grafts have a significantly improved graft survival than those of unmatched grafts. However, the recurrence of the herpes simplex infection is significantly earlier in the HLA-A and -B matched group than in the non- matched group (chapter 10).

Section III

The remaining studies in this thesis addressed themselves to the presence of possible associations between HLA and various ophthalmologic disorders.

General herpes simplex virus infections have a wide distribution in man, but ocular infections with herpes simplex are relatively rare. That fact led us to look for possible deviations in HLA-A, -B, -C and -DR antigen frequencies in a group of patients with recurrent herpes simplex virus keratitis. The frequency of HLA-A3 was significantly elevated in patients with recurrent herpes simplex virus keratitis as compared to healthy controls. Females, especially in the age group 15 to 45, were significantly less affected than males (chapter 11).

HLA-DRw8 is the only significantly elevated DR antigen before correction for the number of antigens studied in herpes simplex virus keratitis patients (chapter 12).

Keratoconus and Fuchs' dystrophy are known as hereditary disorders but sporadic cases occur frequently. Because of the frequently observed familial character of these two diseases, possible associations between the disease and ABO and HLA antigens were studied. There were no significant differences in the ABO and HLA-A, -B and -C antigen frequencies in patients with keratoconus or Fuchs' dystrophy as compared to normal controls. (chapter 13 and 14).

Patients with malignant choroidal melanoma may react against their tumours on an immunological basis (see chapter 15). Since immune responsiveness is coded by genes in the major histocompatibility complex, we analysed the HLA antigen frequencies in patients with malignant choroidal melanoma. A histological subdivision of patients into those with 'pure spindle cell' tumours and those with 'not pure spindle cell' tumours was made because of the differences in their clinical courses and 15 year mortality rates (chapter 15).There was a significant heterogeneity in the frequencyof the HLA-B locus antigens of patients with the 'pure spindle cell' type malignant choroidal melanoma as compared to normal controls, but only borderline heterogeneity in the 'not pure' cell type malignant choroidal melanoma patients. HLA-B27 was significantly different before correction for the number of antigens tested, in those two subsets of malignant choroidal melanoma. It was never present in 35 patients in the 'pure spindle' group and it was present in 5 of the 34 patients in the 'not pure spindle' patients.

A relative excess of blood group O was observed in the 'not pure spindle' cell type malignant choroidal melanoma patients and a relative deficiency of blood group non-O in the 'pure spindle' cell type malignant choroidal melanoma patients.

If the markedly shorter survival times of patients with 'not pure spindle' type of MCM are the results of a relatively reduced immunocompetence associated with blood group O, then those results would be consistent with the hypothesis of Joycey (see chapter 15) that blood group O recipients of renal allografts have prolonged allograft survival times because they are relatively immuno-incompetent as compared to the non-O blood group recipient

Postscript

The chapters 3 to 15 are based on the following acticles:

3. H.J. Völker-Dieben, C.C. Kok-van Alphen and J. D'Amaro. Longterm follow-up study of 19 patients who received 22 corneal grafts between 1939 and 1948 from eyes enucleated because of a malignant choroidal melanoma. Submitted for publication.
4. H.J. Völker-Dieben, C.C. Kok-van Alphen and J. D'Amaro. Survival of 44 corneal grafts obtained from eyes enucleated because of malignant choroidal melanoma. Submitted for publication.
5. H.J. Völker-Dieben, C.C. Kok-van Alphen, Q. Lansbergen and G.G. Persijn (1982) Different influences on corneal graft survival in 539 transplants. Acta Ophthalm. 60: 190-202.
6. H.J. Völker-Dieben, C.C. Kok-van Alphen, Q. Lansbergen and G.G. Persijn (1982) The effect of prospective HLA-A and -B matching on corneal graft survival. Acta Ophthalm. 60: 203-212.
7. H.J. Völker-Dieben, J. D'Amaro, C.C. Kok-van Alphen and P. de Lange. The interactions of HLA-DR, graft size and corneal vascularization of the recipient on graft survival. Submitted for publication.
8. H.J. Völker-Dieben, C.C. Kok-van Alphen and J. D'Amaro. Keratoplasty in children. Submitted for publication.
9. H.J. Völker-Dieben, C.C. Kok-van Alphen and P. de Lange (1984) Corneal grafts for endothelial decompensation: the influence of implant lenses (pseudophakia) on corneal graft survival. Acta Ophthalm. 62: 1-13.
10. H.J. Völker-Dieben, C.C. Kok-van Alphen, J. D'Amaro and P. de Lange (1984) The effect of prospective HLA-A and -B matching in 288 penetrating keratoplasties for herpes simplex keratitis. Acta Ophthalmologica in press.
11. H.J. Völker-Dieben, C.C. Kok-van Alphen, I. Schreuder, J. D'Amaro (1981) HLA-A and -B antigens in recurrent corneal herpes simplex virus infection. Herpetische Augenerkrankungen, p. 91, J.F. Bergmann Verlag, München.

12. H.J. Völker-Dieben and J. D'Amaro. HLA-DR antigens in recurrent corneal herpes simplex virus infection. Submitted for publication.
13. H.J. Völker-Dieben and J. D'Amaro. HLA and ABO antigens in keratoconus patients. Submitted for publication.
14. H.J. Völker-Dieben and J. D'Amaro. HLA and ABO antigens in patients with Fuchs' dystrophy. Submitted for publication.
15. H.J. Völker-Dieben, J. D'Amaro, P. de Lange and D. Wolff-Rouendaal (1983) HLA and ABO antigens in patients with malignant choroidal melanoma. Clin. Exp. Immunol. 53: 581-588

GPSR Compliance

The European Union's (EU) General Product Safety Regulation (GPSR) is a set of rules that requires consumer products to be safe and our obligations to ensure this.

If you have any concerns about our products, you can contact us on ProductSafety@springernature.com

In case Publisher is established outside the EU, the EU authorized representative is:

Springer Nature Customer Service Center GmbH
Europaplatz 3
69115 Heidelberg, Germany

Batch number: 10761599

Printed by Printforce, the Netherlands